CLEAROPATHY

CLEAROPATHY

Dr Solomon Lall

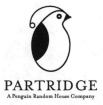

PARTRIDGE

A Penguin Random House Company

To order additional copies of this book, contact
Partridge India
000 800 10062 62
www.partridgepublishing.com/india
orders.india@partridgepublishing.com

I dedicate this book to my loving wife PREETY and my beautiful daughter SARA without whom this would not have been possible.

My sincere thanks to both of them who allow me to do all the community projects I do for the public health and welfare.

CLEAR: *Cellular-biology Level Energy Advancement & Repair*

Clearopathy: A Treatment process which focuses on the Cellular-biology Level Energy Advancement and Repair.

A new branch of Alternate Medicine which uses no modern medicine to cure a number of disorders including FAT LOSS, Weight Loss, STRESS, Depression Obesity, Diabetes, Thyroidism, Impotence, Infertility, PCOS, Sleep Disorders, Cholesterol, Chronic Heart Disorders, Cancer etc. which the present modern day medicines have no answer.

Clearopathy treatment It is a combination of CLEAR process, Psychotherapy, Diet, Nutrition, Fitness and Ayur Assistance

The doctor of the future will give no medicine, but will interest her or his patients in the care of the human frame, in a proper diet, and in the cause and prevention of disease.

Thomas A. Edison
—US inventor (1847-1931)

Introduction and Medical Disclaimer

The book intends to introduce the modern world a branch of Modern Alternate Medicine practice which used no medicne to cure many disorders like FAT LOSS, Weight Loss, STRESS, Depression Obesity, Diabetes, Thyroidism, Impotence, Infertility, PCOS, Sleep Disorders, Cholesterol, Chronic Heart Disorders etc.

This branch of treatment is invented by Dr.

S. LALL

Dr. Lall has been practicing this treatment since last decade.

The material in this book is also intended to provide a review and reflection on the growing concern about the popularity of injesting/taking daily pills/medicine/drugs for every disorder possible.

Taking prescription /non-prescription /over the counter pills for FAT LOSS, Weight Loss, STRESS, Depression Obesity, Diabetes, Thyroidism, Impotence, Infertility, PCOS, Sleep Disorders, Cholesterol, Chronic Heart Disorders etc. or for so many other reasons/ conditions has become a fashion which might result in cancer and many other serious life threatening conditions.

Whereas Emergency Medical Care & Condition warrant and necessitates the use of such medication to save life, **Daily use of these pills** or any sort of chemicals and unnatural pills to resolve any issues without considering the root cause, according to the author **is unwarranted and unnatural**.

Just because these drugs or pills are legally available does not make them less dangerous or life threatening.

The regular consumption of such pills does surely make ordinary people dependent of these drugs and common people become drug addicts without their knowledge and consent.

Most of these drugs do not cure as claimed but control and maintain the problem. This exactly **may not be the outcome** numerous of the **patient around the world actually look for**.

Maintaining a problem would certainly increase the potency of the disorder and with time this disorder will explode and create many more serious health problems.

The author wants common people to use their mind and apply their common senses while taking a decision to become dependent on any such type of unnatural and chemical based pills/medication/drugs for any disorder like FAT LOSS, STRESS, Depression Obesity, Diabetes, Thyroidism, Impotence, Infertility, PCOS, Sleep Disorders, Cholesterol, Chronic Heart Disorders etc.

Popping pills and just forgetting about the disorder and problem is a dream of every individual suffering from various disorders. However no such magic has ever happened in hundred years of Pharmacy medicine.

Nobody likes to think about the cause of these suffering, the real reasons of these disorders. They blind sight themselves and **ignore the "WHY" of the disorder.**

This behavior of Ignorance has become the premise of a very basic psychology, which is exhibited by the whole majority of people suffering from various disorders worldwide.

The memories involved in **the search for reason** is far more painful than popping pills. **The psychological agony of such memories is far more stressful for people.**

Ordinary population of the world just wants to forget the basics of LIFE and rather always finds someone else to blame for their own apathy. A Choice to point out the responsibility of their own health to someone else seems to be the easiest and safest choice.

Shunning ones responsibility towards your own health and wellness is the growing cause of people suffering more and more worldwide.

The author observes that this global phenomenon has crossed all boundaries from rich to poor, and today stands as a cause of concern for general public health. The author feels that the general public should be made aware of.

Steps should be taken to help a larger population. To bring awareness and make common population abstain from drug dependency and make them realize that if they can't take care of their bodies, nobody can.

The author desires to **promote the culture** of people taking responsibility of their own wellbeing instead of blaming any government or non-government agencies or any other authorities worldwide.

Allowing people to Give an opportunity to take responsibility of their own Health can be great step towards protecting Human Species Natural System in future.

Natural Human System's power to Heal by applying Natural and Correctional approach to very common problems and disorders like Diabetes, Thyroidism, PCOS, OBESITY, Infertility, Impotence, Stress and Depression and many more hormonal and immune disorders is the only **Key to Healing**.

The motive of this book is to make people aware that the **Natural correction and natural balance** of human hormone and metabolic system is the natural solution.

It is possible to cure a lot of disorder which become life threatning is not cured for a long time.

The path to cure is available and Clearopathy leads that path.

Balance is the key answer to many problems of human system.

The Correction of hormone imbalance can concurrently correct many of the other common problems like OBESITY, Diabetes, Thyroidism, PCOS, Weight Loss, Infertility, Impotence, Stress, Depression etc.

These simple corrections and act of balance can be of tremendous help to the general population which a great number of common human populations are suffering daily.

Due to such a blind sight a large number of people around the world are dealing with the resultant serious emergent medical conditions daily.

Every effort has been made to provide accurate and dependable information in this book. However, different stream of health-care professionals have differing opinions and advances in every specific domain is humanly impossible to track.

Many outcomes in medical and scientific research are made public very quickly, whereas a large chunk of information never reaches the common people.

Therefore, the publisher, authors, and editors, as well as any other professionals related to this book cannot be held responsible for any error, omission, or dated material.

The author and the publisher do not take any responsibility towards any pain or suffering caused, or feelings of anyone is touched by reading this book.

The intention of the book to share and propagate general misconceptions that can be corrected by any individual who desires better health, wellness. This book is for everyone who would take the responsibilities of their own wellbeing, rather than blame anyone else.

Thus if anyone is not in accordance to the ideas shared is just coincidental and the author and the publisher does not take any responsibilities of such situations and conditions.

This book is not intended as a substitute for the guided health advice of a professional. The reader should regularly consult a related professional in matters relating to his/her health and particularly with respect to any symptoms that may require urgent diagnosis or emergency medical attention.

The author and publisher assume no responsibility for any outcome of applying the information in this book in a program of self-care or under the care of any inexperience and uneducated health practitioner.

Many outcomes in medical and scientific research are made public very quickly, whereas a large chunk of information never reaches the common people.

Therefore, the publisher, authors, and editors, as well as any other professionals related to this book cannot be held responsible for any error, omission, or dated material.

The author and publisher assume no responsibility for any outcome of applying the information in this book in a program of self-care or under the care of any inexperience and uneducated health practitioner.

If you have questions concerning your problems, issues, health, nutrition, diet, fitness, psychology or any information about the application of the any solutions described in this book, consult Dr. Lall's Clearopathy Clinic directly.

As a Psychologist, Nutritionist, Reflexologist, EFT, Ancient Indian Naturopathy, Uropathy expert and a Lifestyle coach for more than a decade, the author have used the concepts outlined in this book for the benefit and welfare of the general public in large numbers.

The author is engaged with a life's commitment to put every effort **to bring this awareness to as many people around the world as possible**, without ever thinking of popularity, marketing or self-promotions.

If you feel you can participate in this effort. Spread the community support project outlined in this book. If you want to start the local community project anywhere in the world contact Dr. Lall's Clinic directly.

"You got Sick in Secret, Now get Healed in a Group Publicly" is a slogan of the Clearopathy Treatment process that you can make popular amongst the common people around the world who desires to get healed.

The same common people **Who are mislead or misinformed about the pills culture.** If you feel same then take steps to **Help large number of people come out of their daily suffering.**

This slogan can be life saving, freedom from medicine, freedom from pain and freedom from suffering for every common individual around the globe. Read more about Dr. Lall's Clearopathy, Attention Abundance Therapy and Freedom from Medicine project in the later Chapter.

Dependency on daily pills is not a class specific disorder. This is not any countries specific disorder. This is not a race, culture or religion specific disorder. **This is human disorder.**

Rich or poor, urban or rural, the disorder and the fallacy in the applications of daily pills/ medicines /drug etc do not spare anyone from its clutches.

If this disorder is not handled responsibly, in less than hundred years of human existence, we will reach a point of No Return.

The complete human population of this Mother Nature earth would be dumped in chemical based support for existence itself.

So **Think** about it rather than finding faults in anyone or pointing fingers at anyone.

Popping Pills is just another popular phenomenon. No one else but we, humans, ourselves are responsible.

The quick fix solution like popping pills, which is so popular and prevalent today is nothing more than our own manifestation of **distorted desires for a quick fix solution**.

We can't just blame the corporations and government for such apathy. Corporations make money that's what they are supposed to do. Governments utilize this to be in power, that's their business.

However general people offering their health of mind and body to such entities are sure fallacy of human population, not of any Corporations or Government.

The cause of concern is the non-application of simple mind and common sense.

The Expectations, that someone else should think about you.

The Hope, that someone else should care about you.

The Desire, that someone else should be responsible for your health and life has blown out of proportions today.

This is psychological disorder which cannot be cured by pills

Certain desires of comfort are good and justified. For instance,

- Someone should stitch your clothes— Considered.
- Someone should build a house for you—Considered.
- Someone should provide the external physical comforts for you—Taken.
- The desire, that someone else should COOK and FEED you—still Granted.

However expecting that someone else should also take the responsibility of your Nutrition, Health and

Hormonal Balance while they FEED you, is a **very dangerous desire, a very dangerous proposition**.

Far more dangerous is expecting that **someone else should heal you with just a pill,** and remove your pains, while you keep damaging yourself on a daily basis without taking any responsibility of your own wellbeing.

The moment you give the authority and responsibility to stuff anything in your mouth or anything that goes into your internal system from your GI Track on a daily basis, **you are trapped.**

Just because you like it doesn't make something good for you. THINK AGAIN.

The DESIRES of physical comforts, if limited to external system can be very beneficial, advancing and comforting.

So what is a solution?

Taking charge, care and responsibility of your internal human system can be a good start.

No matter which state or stage of disorder your mind and body maybe, you might still have a chance **to SAVE YOURSELF.**

If you come out of Your Pills, you might come out of Your Pains.

Let's all contribute to this movement, with whatever minimum efforts possible.

Clearopathy Treatment is **SIMPLE but not EASY.**

Read the book to understand Clearopathy and realize that with a little effort and responsibility towards our own body and physical being, We might have a chance to **SAVE HUMANITY.**

CONTENTS

CHAPTER 1
YOU ALREADY KNOW THIS

> *The mark of your ignorance is the depth of your belief. What the caterpillar calls the end of the world, the Master calls the butterfly.*
>
> —*Richard Bach*

Obesity, Diabetes, Thyroidism, Impotence, Infertility, PCOS, Sleep Disorders, Cholesterol, CHD, etc in America, Australia, UK, India and indeed in many more countries around the world, is reaching epidemic proportions.

As per the reports, more than 65 percent of American and around similar proportions of adults in Australia, UK and India and nearly one-quarter of our children are overweight or obese.

It is not an understatement that obesity is literally killing people around the world, according to various reports America, Australia are leading and setting the stage for a international crisis of cardiovascular disease, diabetes, thyroidism, OBESITY, hypertension, and other related disorders.

The tools for dealing with the health conditions of today are not as specific and precise as those that have been available for the contagious diseases.

Medical science made possible the prevention of the more serious consequences of many of the chronic diseases.

However No specific preventive is available for disorders like obesity STRESS, Depression Obesity, Diabetes, Thyroidism, Impotence, Infertility, PCOS, Sleep Disorders, Cholesterol, Chronic Heart Disorders etc. other than changes in behavioral patterns.

The basic and burning problems of modern style of living all the world over can be listed as under
  (1) Armaments / Nuclear Weapons (Militarism)
  (2) Disturbed Family Relations
  (3) Ecological Pollution
  (4) Tension—Physical, mental, emotional
  (5) Violence and Cruelty
  (6) Corruption / Dishonesty / Immorality
  (7) Drug-Addiction
  (8) Neglect of Law & Order, Ethical, Moral and Social Discipline
  (9) Health Problems—Physical, mental and emotional diseases (including psychosomatic disorders)
  (10) Exploitation

However the **most underlining** problem that **easily loses sight** of any attention is the **growing population living their daily lives totally dependent on chemical**

based pills to manage or control the most important disorder in the human physical system. **The Distortion of neuro-endocrine system.**

The distortion of neuro-endocrine system results in successfully altering the balances and functioning of the hormones dependent on it.

Hormones imbalance eventually results in improper coordination and functioning of the complete body system.

The hormones act as the messenger of good health and balance for the whole body. Any imbalance, harm, pain in the body is notified by the hormones, which in turn switches on the system of the natural healing process through other systems.

Any imbalance to the hormones results eventually in pain, suffering, decay of the body parts associated with its functioning.

While the nervous system coordinates rapid responses to outside stimuli, the endocrine system controls slower, longer-lasting responses to your environment.

The link between these two systems is the hypothalamus, a small, almond-sized gland located in the brain.

Functioning as an endocrine gland, the hypothalamus secretes hormones that stimulate the pituitary gland to release other hormones into the bloodstream.

The pituitary is often referred to as the "master gland," since its hormones act on the thyroid, ovaries, testes, and adrenal glands to regulate growth, reproduction, nutrient absorption, and metabolism.

Basic biology for more than a century had this information. Then Why have mainstream medical research failed so miserably?

Because decade after decade they have continued to look in all the wrong places and wrong direction.

They continue to develop more drugs, all of which are harmful and none of which cure disease.

They continue doing genetic research as though hormonal disorders, cancer and other diseases can be cured by manipulating one's DNA.

But they refuse to study lifestyle factors. They refuse to accept the fact that we give life-threatening disorders & diseases to ourselves by **the way we live, think, act, eat, and handle stress.**

Of course, one main reason they refuse to look at lifestyle factors is that would make all their high-rise glass and metal buildings, their thousands of medical researchers, their Billions of dollars of research funding, and their false erudition, completely irrelevant.

They would have to admit that disorders are caused by one's lifestyle—and therefore can be reversed by changes in one's lifestyle.

However naming these disorders as diseases does open a BIG opportunity for unparallel Business.

Someone has wisely said that the definition of **insanity is doing the same thing over and over again, but expecting a different result.**

That's precisely what Organized Medicine, including the National Health Program of so many countries and nations, has been doing for the last hundred years.

Going down the same research "road" that has failed for decades, yet expecting to have success.

Why doctors are not taught how to get people well from their diseases?

Because the Drug companies have enormous control over medical schools and the training doctors receive because drug companies provide a significant amount of the research funding for medical school research—in large part to develop more drugs! It's the old "golden rule"—"He who has the gold-rules!

Also, drug companies have enormous control over the medical journals and the articles they publish (which establish standards of medical practice) because the medical journals contain more pages of high-priced four-color advertising by the drug companies than actual pages that contain the medical articles.

If a medical journal starts publishing articles that contain information on how to get a patient well without prescribing drugs to the patient, the drug companies will "pull" their expensive advertisements, and that particular medical journal will go bankrupt and cease to exist.

So, it's not hard to figure out why medical journals refuse to publish articles on natural healing, natural medication, natural correction and natural balances.

The food and drink industry has been the muscle of the advertising world. Huge profits are at stake and thus asking people to voluntarily stop junk food would be bad for business.

Conservative estimate suggests that over 60% of the global population could become obese within a generation.

The beverages industry is defensive because of the potential loss in sales and revenues. So they suggest to blame individual for the choice of food. It's much more easier to blame individuals than any particular industry. Business are formed to do business, it an individual choice to eat or not to eat.

Advertising is very much part of our culture and it would over simplistic to say that advertisement do not have any effect on our choices and only through exercise we can lose weight or overcome other issues.

Actually the food industry just does not depend on the necessity to eat drive the market; they actually create the perceived need for food.

The media regulation is proving challenging through the world. The concept of taxing the junk food certainly will also fail.

The industry is against such measure. They prefer things like workout and self control, instead of ban or taxing the business and industry.

The **onus would never taken by the Commercial food Industry.** The preferred alternative to regulation has always been exercise and responsibility of individual to take care of themselves and their choices.

The responsibility is always put on the individual's lack of physical activity and excessive amount of food intake.

When the responsibility shift form the industry to individuals, it becomes easy for business to do business without any guild and costs on the industry,

If industries start taking responsibility they would have to shut down and this would claim competitiveness and jobs from the industry.

Soaring diabetes rates are inextricably tied to the global obesity epidemic. However the Challenge lies in the lack of political will of the various governments of the world to change certain cultural habits and to take on powerful industries promoting such habits that lead to these problems.

From 1970 to 1990 the first onset of obesity was experienced by our world. The obesity epidemic started mainly due to the decline of physical activity.

It was commonly believed and perceived that we have less time to do things, however in reality we were spending more time in front of our television sets and leading and inactive life.

Later this obesity epidemic was propelled by the increase in food consumption. The increase supply of food at lower cost was matched with the increase in the appetite or the people and the inactive lifestyle.

Supersizing of food portions accelerated the process. This reflected the failure of the free market that demands government intervention.

Today the commercial market has a wide variety of foods that are actually unhealthy but are very successfully marketed to kids. These foods get special mention in the children section as the best food for children, making obesity not an easy challenge to overcome in time to come.

Many innovative and extremely attractive resources are deployed to support that industry which cannot remain untouched by children and youth of the day.

The recognition that prevention strategies is more important to contain the obesity epidemic is the missing link and the unequal distribution is the consequence of the complex system on how our society manages its affairs.

Suitable steps must be taken to tackles the inequities in the system. The imbalance in the distrituion of ample and nutrition global and national food supplies. Create environments that themselves make eas the access and uptake of healtheir option.

Living and working condition can produce more equual material and mental resources between and in the social group

This will require action at local, national and global levels.

Other issues and problems that stand out include:
- Encouraging/advertising unhealthy diets and foods (especially to children);
- Generally putting low priority on health;
- Industry-dominated food policy at the expense of local grocery stores;
- Deteriorating health of children in poverty; and so on.

Childhood obesity is associated with a higher chance of premature death and disability in adulthood.

The WHO adds, "What is not widely known is that the risk of health problems starts when someone is only very slightly overweight, and that the likelihood of problems increases as someone becomes more and more overweight.

Many of these conditions cause long-term suffering for individuals and families. In addition, the costs for the health care system can be extremely high."

With obesity comes increasing risks of
- Cardiovascular disease
- Diabetes (type 2)
- Musculoskeletal disorders.
- Cancers.

According to The WHO that many low-and middle-income countries are now facing a "double burden" of disease:

- While they continue to deal with the problems of infectious disease and under-nutrition, at the same time they are experiencing a rapid upsurge in chronic disease risk factors such as obesity and overweight.
- It is now common to find under-nutrition and obesity existing side-by-side within the same country, the same community and even within the same household.

- This double burden is caused by inadequate pre-natal, infant and young child nutrition followed by exposure to high-fat, energy-dense, micronutrient-poor foods and lack of physical activity.

For the first time in human history, the number of overweight people is competing head to head with the number of underweight people . . . . While the world's underfed population has declined slightly since 1981 to 1.2 billion, the number of overweight people has surged to 1.3 billion.

- The population of overweight people has grown rapidly in recent decades, more than the health gains from the modest decline in hunger.
- In the United States, 65 percent of adults are overweight by international standards. A whopping 43 percent of American adults are considered obese. And the trend is spreading to children as well, with one in five American kids now classified as overweight.
- Obesity cost the United States 12 percent of the national health care budget in the late 1990s, $118 billion, more than double the $47 billion attributable to smoking.
- Overweight and obesity are advancing rapidly in the developing world as well. While 80 percent of the world's hungry children live in countries with food surpluses.
- Techno-fixes like liposuction or olestra attract more attention than the behavioral patterns

like poor eating habits and sedentary lifestyles that underlie obesity.

- Liposuction is now the leading form of cosmetic surgery in the United States, for example, at 400,000 operations per year. While billions are spent on gimmicky diets and food advertising, far too little money is spent on nutrition education. Same is phenomenon is trending all over the globe.

—**Chronic Hunger and Obesity Epidemic; Eroding Global Progress, World Watch Institute, March 4, 2000**

Childhood obesity is also an increasing concern for the WHO:
- The problem [of childhood obesity] is global and is steadily affecting many low-and middle-income countries, particularly in urban settings.
- Globally, in 2010 the number of overweight children under the age of five, is estimated to be over 42 million. Close to 35 million of these are living in developing countries.
- Overweight and obese children are likely to stay obese into adulthood and more likely to develop non-communicable diseases like diabetes and cardiovascular diseases at a younger age.

—*Childhood overweight and obesity, WHO, last accessed August 22, 2010*

Obesity Affects Poor as well as Rich
Obesity also affects the poor as well, due to things like marketing of unhealthy foods

"Restrictions in access to food determine two simultaneous phenomena that are two sides of the same coin: poor people are malnourished because they do not have enough to feed themselves, and they are obese because they eat poorly, with an important energy imbalance. The food they can afford is often cheap, industrialized, mass produced, and inexpensive."

- 33.4 million living with HIV
  Within this whole fiasco of health problems there is a huge population of people who really goes unnoticed.
- This population has a desire to be healthy and want to cure themselves.
- This population is present in almost every part of the globalized world.
- This population consists of people who are on daily pills to fight various disorders.
- They depend on prescription on non-prescription drugs to tackle various type of human disorders they are diagnosed with.
- This population, relentlessly trust anyone who can suggest them quick fix to their health problems.
- Their pains and suffering is being just delayed by a pill.
- This is the population of people who are absolutely unaware of the consequences of

the culture of taking chemically based pills for medication.

We allocate high priest status to doctors and we abdicate our own responsibility to look after our own health.

Such behaviors have led to the invention and growth of the real-time monitoring technological, such technology monitoring of our bodies is likely to become a reality.

There is a deeper level of pathology to this, than our pill culture; **a step further away from knowing and achieving real health.**

The fact is, we are all able to easily monitor our own health by simply sensing it or, better, "feeling" it. But we disregard it.

Homo sapiens appear to be the only species on the planet that seems confused about how to sense and seek health.

The origin of the pill culture and the techno-health culture lies in a **disease-oriented culture**, while these distractions are largely circumvented with a health-oriented culture.

The pendulum has swung much too far. Over the past few decades, we've gone from being reluctant to recognize and treat any diagnosis to a populations addicted to the quick fix, whether there's a real problem or not.

Practitioners are handing out medicine pills like it's party candy, and perfectly healthy young men, women and children, be they the college student are becoming addicted to stimulants with tragic consequences. And it's all under the aegis of legitimate medical practice.

What is interesting that the pills ruining so many lives, are distributed and sanctioned by the medical community, based on "diagnostic tests" that are so loose they would be laughable if the results weren't so dire.

Detailed diagnoses and long term treatment just don't pay, and our microwave culture demands the short-cut solution of a pill, despite that research is only just beginning to show the harmful, long-term results of pill used by individuals.

Layer onto this the tremendous amount of advertising dollars that are being poured into promoting pill treatments for adults and children.

Fat Loss, Obesity, Thyroid pills has become a norm amongst women. Every other woman I meet has at least been taking some sort of pills.

We have become a Global human population of pill-poppers who use drugs to beat aches and pains instead of changing their diet and lifestyle

Students use pills that are classified as a class-A drug which has an effect similar to cocaine and speed on healthy adults—to help them cram for exams and work through study crises,

One of the most interesting aspects of the rise of drug culture is the way it has marginalized psychological explanation. It used to be thought that peptic ulcers, for example, were caused by stress and anxiety, or being screwed up by your parents.

But today, whatever your problem, there's bound to be a drug for it nowadays: something to perk you up, clear your complexion, relive from common headache, simple pains, sleep, revitalize your sex life, etc.

Think of the number of people who order Viagra over the internet not because they suffer from impotence but because they're curious about the extra kick the drug will give their love life.

Now there is an acid-suppressant drug that relieves symptoms. To take the staggeringly obvious example, Viagra has sidelined the whole idea of sexual counseling, because whether your problem is medical, quasi-medical or psychological, Viagra does the business.

Nobody even put a bit of mind about the serious consequences of exposing their internal body system to such potent and dangerous chemicals.

Let us consider few of the popular and widely used pills world over.

Thyroid Pills
Daily Thyroid pills is one the most common pills taken by women around the world and all that I have come across in the last decade.

For every other hormonal disorder discovered in women, women around the world are popping the pills as if it's some secret magic recipe.

For women around I openly state: **It's not your fault. You are led to believe with so much conviction and excellent marketing that your hormones are damaged, the only way out is pills".**

For a female the word hormone is very sacred. They may or may not understand the human hormone but You talk hormone and they are all heads up. This made thyroid pills become popular faster than anti-pregnancy pills. The marketing data reveals it all. More women take thyroid pills than any other pills around the world and no one ever bothers to question such pill culture.

The marketing around such pills has been so powerful and so effective that no ordinary person stands a chance. Everybody wants a better and safe life and if only daily pills are supposed to do, then why not they think.

Taking replacement thyroid hormones pills without addressing the underlying immune imbalance is doomed to fail.

Yet By misrepresenting, a shoddy, poorly researched and misguided opinion piece as analysis, capped by a panicky headline.

Many health and pharmacy professionals are also veering away from their purported mission of helping patients educate and protect themselves, instead proposing that patients to get into a lifelong dependency of thyroid drug **that may not work all to cure but to maintain the disorder.**

The ultimate effect of hypothyroidism, whether it's caused by iodine deficiency or autoimmunity, is to decrease the amount of thyroid hormone available to the body naturally.

Most people are unaware that hypothyroidism is an autoimmune disease and this is one of the main reasons why **conventional pharmaceutical treatments are ineffective** for more than 80 percent of patients with sluggish thyroids.

Diabetes Pills
The Type II diabetes diagnostics is one the largest contributor to the daily pills culture.

Type 2 diabetes means the body has a problem with insulin. This causes blood sugar to get too high. **Insulin**

is a hormone, or chemical, made by the body that is needed to change food into energy.

When you have type 2 diabetes, your body either does not make enough insulin, or it doesn't use insulin as well as it should.

Diabetes is not treated but very commonly controlled or maintained at controlled levels with insulin or oral medicines (pills)

People with type 2 diabetes are unable to properly break down carbohydrates, either because their bodies do not produce enough insulin or because they've become resistant to the hormone, which controls blood sugar levels.

These patients are at higher risk for heart attacks, kidney problems, blindness and other serious complications.

Many diabetics require multiple drugs with different mechanisms of action to control their blood sugar levels.

Type 2 diabetes medications can prevent dangerous blood sugar levels, **but can also be harmful by themselves.**

Some diabetes drugs, however, comes with severe side effects, including hypoglycemia, bladder cancer, lactic acidosis, acute pancreatitis and cardiac problems.

Hypoglycemia can be caused by pills, which work to control blood sugar by stimulating the pancreas to release insulin. Hypoglycemia from some pills can be long-lasting and very dangerous.

Symptoms of hypoglycemia are increased heartbeat; sweating; paleness; anxiety; numbness in fingers, toes and lips; sleepiness; confusion; headache and slurred speech.

Bladder cancer has been tied to another very common diabetic pill. It works by helping the body cells use insulin and reducing the amount of glucose released by the liver.

Unfortunately, the world's best-selling diabetes drug is also among the most dangerous. Studies show that a patient has a 40 percent increased risk of developing bladder cancer if this diabetic is taken for more than a year

Users can experience other side effects, as well, including vision problems, weakened bones and heart problems.

Symptoms of bladder cancer are an increased need to urinate, pain during urination and discoloration or blood in the urine.

Lactic acidosis has been reported as a rare side effect of another diabetic pill, which work by reducing the amount of glucose produced by the liver. Lactic acidosis occurs when lactic acid builds up in the bloodstream and oxygen levels in the body drop.

Symptoms of lactic acidosis are nausea and weakness. Blood tests that measure electrolyte levels should be conducted during the first few weeks of taking any drug in this family of chemical formulation.

Acute pancreatitis can be caused by GLP-Inhibitors, which increase insulin secretion in the pancreas. The sudden inflammation of the pancreas can be life-threatening.

Symptoms of acute pancreatitis are intense stomach pain, nausea and vomiting. Cardiac problems have been associated with many class of diabetic pills. These include heart attacks, which can be fatal.

Symptoms of heart failure include swelling in the legs or ankles, gaining a lot of weight in a short time, difficulty breathing, coughing and fatigue.

While there's little you can do to prevent developing type 1 diabetes. Its number one risk factor is genetic, you have control over most risk factors for type 2 diabetes.

Just about anyone can develop type 2 diabetes, but research has identified characteristics that make you more susceptible to the disease. Here they are, broken into two categories: those you cannot control, and those you can.

Diabetes Risk Factors You Cannot Control
First, the bad news. There are some type 2 diabetes risk factors that you simply cannot control. They include:

Genetics. Some research has found that people who have been diagnosed with type 2 diabetes typically have at least one close relative with the disease.

Age. Most people with type 2 diabetes (diagnosed and undiagnosed) are age 20 or older, with the highest percentage falling in the 60-and-older age group. Most cases recently have emerged for the population falling in the age 39-55 years old.

Ethnicity. Statistics show that diabetes is more common in African Americans, Latinos, Native Americans, Asian, and Pacific Islanders. However this doesn't exclude other population from the risk with today's lifestyle and food choices.

Diabetes Risk Factors You Can Control
You may not be able to change your age, ethnicity, and genetic makeup, but you have significant control over the remaining risk factors for type 2 diabetes. That's because they are overwhelmingly associated with lifestyle.

Diet & Nutrition. What you eat has a profound effect on your blood glucose levels and your risk of developing blood sugar problems. A diet high in starches, sugars, and other high-glycemic carbohydrates only leads to weight gain but also decreases insulin sensitivity. These composition of food rapidly break down into glucose and drive up blood sugar levels, and you significantly increase your risk.

Weight. One of the most significant risk factors for type 2 diabetes is obesity. Statistics show that 90 percent of all people with type 2 diabetes are overweight. Where you store those extra pounds is also an issue. If you carry them in the abdominal area, you are at an even greater risk of insulin resistance and type 2 diabetes.

That's because abdominal fat is more metabolically active than fat stored in the hips or buttocks. It is more easily broken down into free fatty acids that enter the bloodstream, interfere with the action of insulin, and raise triglyceride and glucose levels. Fortunately, losing weight often is all it takes to lower the risk of type 2 diabetes.

Activity level. Lack of regular exercise lowers insulin sensitivity and increases the possibility of metabolic syndrome, another type 2 diabetes risk factor.

Alcohol & Smoking. Everyone knows that smoking increases your risk of cancer, but many probably don't know that people who smoke are at increased risk of developing high blood pressure—which can make them more susceptible to type 2 diabetes.

Prescription drugs. Drugs that increase your risk of developing type 2 diabetes include corticosteroids (typically prescribed to treat asthma and arthritis); thiazide diuretics (often used to treat heart failure and high blood pressure); and beta blockers (drugs used to treat hypertension).

Obesity and FAT LOSS/ Weight LOSS Pills
The best and the fastest selling pills, around the world are weight loss pills. People pick this pill through prescription, over the counter and even secretly.

This pills come under the category of weight management. The weight loss pills industry is a very large industry and commercially very successful.

Obesity has not been given an epidemic status though a large number of countries around the globe have surpassed the fifty percent mark.

It is correct, Obesity cannot be called because epidemic as it is not a communicable disease, and neither does it have any immediate threat to life. In fact obesity is good for economy for so many countries and so many business of the world.

Today's Good economy depends on more consumption everything. Be it food or any other material.

More consumption, more sales, better economy and again at the same time more sick people so more sales of medications pills for all the disease and disorder that follow the obesity.

This cycle is hugely successful for economy.

There is no cure or medication for obesity and thus it cannot be a labeled as medical emergency.

However many general population fails to understand if you let your bodies become overweight or obese. It is not normal. It may come as a surprise that just a few decades ago, obesity was not considered as normal, whereas today it's been accepted as normal.

People who become overweight start to believe in the popular misconception that reduction in calories would reverse their overweight problem.

Most fail to understand, overweight is initially just a symptom.

These symptoms are normally due to the imbalances in hormones caused due to improper and incorrect ingestion of food which the body could not metabolize to produce the life substance to maintain a healthy body.

When the initial attempts of starvation fail to give results, overweight people try all sorts of fad diets, which do not last.

These overweight individuals secretly then turn towards an easy fix again and that is : "diet pills" which eventually graduates to taking FAT loss pills along with some or many other unnatural chemical based substance, just to lose weight.

The combination of popular and fat diets, diet pills, fat loss pills and other substance abuse leads to disaster to the already batter hormone system. The hormone system gets a nose dive down into total chaos.

By this time the overweight individual has already entered into the obesity domain. Then they realize that have lost their battles with weight loss.

They start blaming everything around and eventually forget that they continued looking for quick fixes all their life.

Their desires to seek quick fix, and their attitude resulted in a situation which went out of control. This continues, till this situation converts into some serious medical condition, requiring bigger and greater medical attention and weight loss steps aside and medical disorder takes priority.

Weight loss pills, be it medically prescribed, natural, herbal or by any other name can be dangerous. The dangers of FAT Loss pills and other Weight Loss pills can be horrifying. The result is the total imbalance in your natural hormonal balance.

Natural herbal diet pills carry much the same risk as prescription or other diet pills do. In fact, some can even be more dangerous.

If you are currently taking weight loss pills, or are even considering taking them, then **you should be aware of the dangers of taking these pills.**

Few of the dangers are listed below for ready reference :
- ➢ increased heart rate
- ➢ heart functions irregularities
- ➢ gastrointestinal disorders
- ➢ stomach irritation
- ➢ nervousness
- ➢ increase blood pressure
- ➢ cause dry mouth
- ➢ cause constipation
- ➢ cause insomnia
- ➢ headache
- ➢ diarrhea
- ➢ high blood pressure
- ➢ irritability
- ➢ stroke
- ➢ heart attack
- ➢ addiction
- ➢ undesirable interactions with other prescription drugs/pills you are taking
- ➢ Long term damage and disruption to natural hormones and hormone imbalance
- ➢ Constant stimulation through pills can change the body's ability to regulate itself and its weight.
- ➢ With constant and long term use of such pills, cancer and other serious health issues, even death.

There are literally hundreds of pills in this category, and they may of may not be regulated at all. This means you really do not know what you are getting when you buy or pop these pills. Many of the companies make false claims that are too good to be true and carry huge risks!

More and more obese people are left to believe that being overweight or obese is normal, and slogans like accept yourself, be proud of yourself even when you are obese, do not listen to anyone, you are not alone become a popular wisdom of all individuals who are suffering.

Yes, by and large, the authorities responsible to create awareness on issues related to obesity have failed, Opening door for road side vendors claiming a new magic pill for weight loss or fat loss every other day. Major Corporation in the world depends on people to be confused and mislead about obesity.

Obesity is **not just a food problem**. It's the choice and composition of the choice of food which is problematic. Food combination or the chemical combination of the food which does not adapted or adjust to the internal system of your body. Incorrect food combination creates Imbalances.

Food is nothing but natural chemical containing Carbon, Hydrogen, Oxygen, Ammonia, Nitrogen etc. These are chemical atoms and molecules in different forms and formats combined together. These are studied in the Organic Chemistry. These natural organic chemical react and fuse with the Biological system of the human body.

There is a science of Biology which governs the internal human system which still remains unexplored to a very large extent. Just identifying and naming parts of organ. Defining their certain functions does not contribute to the science of biology. It's just the beginning.

When dealing with obesity the most common mistake that has been promoted since decades is the application of Physical principals of Thermodynamic.

This according to me is one of the biggest fallacies of medical science and general popular culture.

How can you forget the basic biology and adapt to the physical principal of thermodynamics before you correct the biological functions of the human body. How can you even not consider the internal chemical reaction and biological interaction of cell in the human system?

Calorie in = Calorie out is the one BIGGEST MISTAKE in modern world which is hindering in the fight against obesity.

Just because someone became famous using such statement doesn't make this statement scientifically true and beneficial for the whole populations.

Every street vendor and so called fitness expert without the basic knowledge of biology or organic chemistry have started giving tips and secrets of losing fat, **when none of them actually have understood the simple question "WHY" it happens.**

Within the human body system, Nothing happen in Isolation. So how a single basic principle of Physics taught in class III can be applied to such a complex situation of obesity and weight loss.

Medical science is the stream which was developed on the principle of studying sick and diseased human body. Even till today, so much about the human body and mind system is not even understood by medical science.

A lot has happened in the last 200 years in the area of medical science, which the common population has no idea. The common populations have no idea who controls or governs the so called information in medical science.

How the advances of early medicine which were focused on cure has been diverted and hijacked into medicine which makes people sick and dependent throughout their lives.

The advancement in medical science and the understanding in human care were much stronger prior to 1940 than it is today.

So many basic principles of medical science which were focused on cure, tried to **answer the question WHY.** This was the status of medical science prior to the world war.

After that what happened is rarely known or spoken about in any major media, discussion, schools or universities.

However after the world war much of which is known today as modern medical science is focused on maintaining the status, controlling it from becoming worse after diagnosis.

Certainly CURE is not one of the objectives of modern medicine.

One of the prominent examples is comparing the advance in the technology utilized in warfare and weapons, airplanes and mechanics included and the advancement in the treatment of cancer.

The status of explanation about cancer and the methods of treatment have not changed since 1948. It's only made available to larger population.

What advancement we have seen in one area of destruction is nowhere seen with cancer research or cure. This is just one of the examples from many.

Physical science will align itself when the basic building block of human biology and its interaction with the system is in balance to the natural state of human body.

WHY fat accumulates in human cell is more important to understand before taking any steps to fight the fat out your body.

Many popular magazines and main stream media is governed and operated by the least of educated people in science.

Popularity is usually the parameter for anything that hits people.

In the quick fix world, the media tries to provide everything that sells. Since many decades media was just a catalyst for misinformation and chaos in the area of health care and wellness.

Issue like Lipophilia was known to German and Austrian doctor prior to 1940, but not today. Neither do they ever care to know it today.

The hormonal imbalance is reason for so many disorders. Obesity is one of them.

Why hormonal imbalance happens suddenly to someone who has been healthy and fine for the 1st thirty years of their live. It's very simple; it takes a long time to actually naturally distort your body balance.

Continuous use of natural chemical substance i.e. food, which is high in starch or simple carbohydrates, specially specified into higher Glycemic Index group or any food substance that increases the insulin level in your body quickly.

Any food combination that spikes the insulin in your blood system can trigger an imbalance.

Besides Accidents and Deadly communicable disease, Human internal body system does not reacts or responds so suddenly to become a disorder.

It takes years and years of abuse "To create huge disorder".

Majority of population since the day a human is born, a continuous imbalanced intake of food create the platform for major disorder later in life.

What is the most basic need for our body is the least of our interest.

While dealing with disorders, the popular science very heavily focuses on exceptions to create a Rule.

What is not natural is focused and the need of correction or avoidance is thrown to a large population or people who might not even be related to such disorders.

The vicious cycle that leads to type 2 diabetes

Insulin resistance is one of the biggest causes of type 2 diabetes. But what causes insulin resistance?

The answer is obesity.

Insulin resistance and obesity go hand in hand. In fact, each problem makes the other worse—which is why it's so important to lose weight if you want to overcome insulin resistance and type 2 diabetes.

Why Insulin Resistance Is Worse When You're Overweight
Obesity simply throws fuel on the fire. Adipose tissue—otherwise known as fat, especially in the abdominal area—releases fatty acids that impair beta-cell function and insulin sensitivity.

It also produces immune cells that lead to chronic, low-grade inflammation. Inflammation also increases insulin resistance and the risk of type 2 diabetes.

Fat cells also secrete hormones, including the hormone leptin. **Leptin is best known for its role in appetite and energy metabolism.** However, research has recently shown that it also has direct effects on insulin secretion and beta-cell growth.

How Insulin Resistance Drives Up Weight
At the same time, the high insulin levels that are characteristic of type 2 diabetes promote weight gain. That's because insulin is the body's primary fat-storage hormone.

As it's working to get glucose into the cells, it's also storing fat. So, the higher your insulin level, the greater your potential of weight gain.

The bottom line: If you want to minimize your insulin resistance and prevent type 2 diabetes, you simply must get a handle on your weight.

Again Pills are not the answer. The only way to reduce insulin level in your body is to seek permanent solution wherein your body system is tuned to produce balanced insulin naturally for proper body functioning.

FAT LOSS Pills or Weight LOSS Pills might actually be disturbing other hormonal balance.

Pills are temporary quick fix and the result is greater damage to the system in the long run. The damage becomes dangerous with continued pumping of the chemical pills.

Only Natural correction through nutrition can make this balance possible and give the power back to the body to manage insulin levels conducive to the normal body functioning and balance the hormone system in the body.

BP & Cholesterol Pills
From the inception of the diet-heart hypothesis in the early 1950s, those who argued that dietary fat caused heart disease accumulated the evidential equivalent of a mythology to support their belief.

These myths are still passed on faithfully to the present day.

According to them this over-nutrition was certainly the cause of obesity. Eating too many calories was the problem, and since fat contains more than twice as many calories per gram as either protein or carbohydrates, "people who cut down on fat usually lose weight," as the Washington Post reported in 1985.

A healthy diet, by definition, **had suddenly** become a low-fat diet.

By following the Medical knowledge, which in dominantly controlled or guided by the Modern American Medical System, throughout the world, the incidence of obesity and diabetes increased and is still increasing at an alarming rate.

The surge in obesity and diabetes occurred as the population was being bombarded with the message that dietary fat is dangerous and that carbohydrates are good for the heart and for weight control.

Foods lower in dietary fat became higher in carbohydrates and people ate more. The result has been a polarization on the subject of nutrition.

Most people still believe that saturated fat, if not any and all fat, is the primary dietary evil. According to them butter, fat, cheese, nuts and eggs will clog our arteries and put on weight. So they have reduced their intakes.

Public-health experts and many in the media continue to insist that the obesity epidemic means the

population doesn't take their advice and continues to shun physical activity while eating fatty foods to excess.

Cholesterol itself is a pearly-white fatty substance that can be found in all body tissues, an essential component of cell membranes and a constituent of a range of physiologic processes, including the metabolism of human sex hormones.

Cholesterol is also a primary component of atherosclerotic plaques, so it was a natural assumption that the disease might begin with the abnormal accumulation of cholesterol. Proponents of the hypothesis then envisioned the human circulatory system as a kind of plumbing system.

Stamler referred to the accumulation of cholesterol in lesions (*A region in an organ or tissue that has suffered damage.*) on the artery walls as "biological rust" that can "spread to choke off the flow of blood, or slow it just like rust inside a water pipe so that only a dribble comes from your faucet."

This imagery is so compelling that we still talk and read about artery-clogging fats and cholesterol, as though the fat of a greasy hamburger were transported directly from stomach to artery lining.

What kept the cholesterol hypothesis particularly viable through the years was that any physician could measure cholesterol levels in human subjects.

Correctly interpreting the measurements was more difficult.

A host of phenomena will influence cholesterol levels, some of which will also influence our risk of heart disease: exercise, for instance, lowers total cholesterol. Weight gain appears to raise it; weight loss, to lower it temporarily.

Cholesterol levels will fluctuate seasonally and change with body position. **Stress will raise cholesterol.** Male and female hormones will affect cholesterol levels, as will diuretics, sedatives, tranquilizers, and alcohol.

For these reasons alone, our cholesterol levels can change by 20 to 30 percent over the course of weeks

Dietary cholesterol, for instance, has an insignificant effect on blood cholesterol. It might elevate cholesterol levels in a small percentage of highly sensitive individuals, but for most of us, it's clinically meaningless.

In science, researchers often evoke a drunk-in-the-streetlight metaphor to describe such situations: One night a man comes upon a drunk crawling on hands and knees on the pavement under a streetlight.

When the man asks the drunk what he's doing, the drunk says that he's looking for his keys. "Is this where you lost them?" asks the man. "I don't know where I lost them," says the drunk, "but this is where the light is." **For the past half-century, cholesterol was where the light was.**

The evolution of medical science after the world wars has suffered enormously, although sometimes unavoidably, by the degree of specialization needed to make progress. "Each science confines itself to a fragment of the evidence and weaves its theories in terms of notions suggested by that fragment.

This problem is clearly exhibited in the study of nutrition, obesity, and chronic disease because significant observations emerge from so many diverse disciplines.

Patient who have been diagnosed with higher level of LDL cholesterol are suggested to take pills for about a year by the medical doctor, come to me for guidance.

When my clinic offers them to take balance dietary and essential fat, they raise their eyebrows with surprise and suspicion initially.

They share their fears that according to their common knowledge, food such as nuts are considered to be fatty and cholesterol laden, how come it's going to bring their cholesterol to normal level.

Such questions and many similar queries like these propel me to tell them the story behind low fat diet hypothesis which is responsible for their imbalanced conditions.

Only Natural correction through nutrition make these patients get back to their balanced levels of Cholesterol within weeks and months of proper guidance. Most of my patients do not even take a single pill to normalize.

PCOS, Birth Control Pills, Infertility Pills and any other Menstrual cycle altering Pills for Women

In my practice I have come across many women who approached a medical practitioner requesting for early or delayed cycles for some reasons.

A very simple fix is handed over to these women in the form of a pill, which these women without any reluctance pop into their system, never realizing how much harm they are inflicting to the natural hormonal balance and systems.

It is surprising and frustrating to see that most doctor feel that the first line of defense against PCOS is the birth control pill.

Millions of women worldwide take the Pill to regulate their cycle, and many of them start in their teens.

According to a recent survey, one third of teens ages 15 to 19 are on the Pill solely for non-contraceptive reasons, such as cysts and missed periods.

It is important to remember that there is no instant pill to make the PCOS symptoms go away.

For **PCOS**, If you are currently taking the Pill or are thinking about it, here are some risk factors to consider:
- Increased insulin resistance
- Increase risk of heart attack or stroke
- The Pill lowers levels of valuable nutrients
- The Pill lowers libido
- In-fertility threats
- The Pill can kill off friendly bacteria in your gut

The pill merely masking the symptoms and in turn, was make the underlying cause (insulin resistance) worse.

Your hypoglycemia can go out of control, **You can gain weight, might lose your sex drive, become frigid, etc.**

Up to 70 percent of women with PCOS are also insulin-resistant, which can scramble your mix of sex hormones even more.

Plus, insulin resistance may increase the risk for type 2 diabetes, heart disease and—if you do manage to get pregnant-complications such as gestational diabetes and preterm labor.

Don't discount the value of having a regular monthly cycle to help prevent uterine cancer, but you can regulate your cycles focused nutrition & workout and natural food ingredients to back your cycle to normalcy.

Some of the common risks of **Birth Control Pills**
- bloating,
- weight gain,

- headaches and fatigue.
- potential blood clots.
- lowered libido,
- headaches,
- breast tenderness,
- mood swings
- menstrual spotting
- other uncomfortable common side effects,
- increase blood clots,
- risk of future infertility
- breast cancer risk and risk of liver tumors.

Risk of **Fertility pills**/drugs/medication etc.
- risk of multiples (twins, triplets and High Order Pregnancies) when using fertility drugs.
- risk that comes with fertility drug use is ovarian hyperstimulation syndrome (OHSS) OHSS can be life-threatening
- Risk to estrogen levels
- Drug Reaction to the pills like Hot flushes, feeling down or irritable, headaches and restlessness.
- Ectopic pregnancy (An embryo implants outside the uterus.)
- The risk of birth defects

Menstrual cycle altering Pills

Women get into altering of menstrual cycle for cultural and social reasons, do not realize the dangers of playing with Mother Nature. Menstruation is an integral part of womanhood.

A pill that suppresses it essentially defines normal menstruation as a problem, potentially leading to a negative body image.

Doctors may not openly support the idea of menstrual suppression only but are rarely reluctant to prescribe when asked.

These pills besides the obvious are not without some common risks :

Those risks include blood clots, stroke, breast tenderness, nausea and headaches, to name a few, For women who also smoke, the risks are even greater.

The effects on bone health, heart health, cancer risks, and fertility are all known. There are also additional concerns with regard to adolescent girls and young women who put off menstruation while their bodies are still maturing.

The kind of pain and suffering these women go in later year of their life is never discussed nor propagated through popular media because it bad for medical and pharma business

Some women like the idea of using hormones to control their cycles and suppress their periods.

The health implications and long-term effects of continuous or extended hormonal contraception use can create total hormonal imbalance and chaos in the natural health of a woman's endocrine and reproductive system.

In the world of health and fitness, every other woman who undergoes treatment at my clinic, one question I routinely ask them, is about the kind of pregnancy they have undergone and the answer from majority comes as C-section/caesarian.

Today caesarian has become the norm, women respond and approach caesarian with so much conviction **as if children were never born naturally prior to the concept of caesarian.**

It has come to a point in today's world, whoever can afford the pay or is covered medically are either pushed to caesarian or willingly chose this method as the only method of delivery amongst women.

I let the common population take their own decision to understand for a moment what exactly we are thinking and what exactly are we doing when we let our women undergo such threatening situations during the most important experience of her life.

The most beautiful experience becomes the worst nightmare for so many women around the world.

In the name of health and wellness, I see females starving themselves to dire consequences. Without any strength they go ahead with labor and child birth and then expect a doctor to take care.

In such situation when women fail to take care of themselves for any reason, and undergo pregnancy, during the child birth the choice for the medical practitioner becomes so obvious.

Operate, cut and take out the baby, because the woman in question doesn't have the strength to deliver the baby naturally.

Most of you might be aware and thus what am I about to tell you a very typical statement in any language in any country all around the world which remains same or similar, kindly pay attention to this statement which I have heard so frequently nowadays . . .

The concerned medical practitioner involved in the process to assist the child birth for women would say **"You have to allow caesarian or else the life of mother and child is in danger"**

Which family on earth would go against such suggestion at the last moment ? at such a critical moment.

Today all who can afford to pay and in other cases those who are insured medically would never deny a **request which is presented with a threat of two lives.**

NO CHOICE. Its a lose lose situation for the women In labor and a win win situation for the concerned medical practitioner.

Understanding the importance of hormonal balance since childhood and taking all natural steps to keep it strong. Not playing around with Pills, would save millions of women who suffer and are traumatized throughout their lives.

Impotency Pills / Erectile dysfunction Pill for Men

- Medically prescribed, natural or herbal pills all pose similar risks like headache, facial flushing, nasal congestion, diarrhea, backache, blue vision cardiac abnormalities
- men with cardiovascular disorder this can be live threatening
- The problem is their effect on arteries. All arteries, not just those in the penis, generate nitric oxide, so any artery can widen in response to impotency pills, causing blood pressure to drop temporarily by 5-8 mmHg, even in healthy men.

Organic nitrates are drugs that widen arteries by increasing their supply of nitric oxide; that's how they open the partially blocked coronary arteries in patients with angina.

Threat of heart attach, strokes is common for men with a history of congestive heart failure or unstable angina, and in men with low blood pressure or uncontrolled high blood pressure

Impotency pills may interact in dangerous ways with drugs that a consumer is already taking, People with diabetes, high blood pressure, high cholesterol, or heart disease are often prescribed drugs containing nitrates, and men with these conditions commonly suffer from ED,

There is no better alternative than revitalizing and giving back the body the strength that mother nature provides through the nutrition available in daily food, you should only know how to choose and use it.

People having ED and other impotency or infertility, should not hesitate to contact Dr. Lall's Nature Care Clinic rather than do senseless things and mess up your physical and psychological balance.

Stop falling prey to the same tricks used over and over by all kind of street side vendor to fool men with ED all around the world.

Sleep Disorders Pills
One of the very basic requirement of the healthy body and the balance of natural cycle is SLEEP. Most of the growth hormones as secreted and do their work of healing the wear and tear of the human system, both physical and psychological.

The problem of the day, this most important natural process itself is in danger for so many of the people globally.

Right through the advent and utilization of unnatural light to extend our day, the consequence has been emerging slow but surely. Today the consequence have taken enormous form and proportions. Sleep disorder is one of these consequences which has now reached our teen age human population.

Places on earth where people are bound by nature to sleep after the sunset rarely come across something like SLEEP Disorder.

Think before you pop a pill to Sleep. The pill does not give you Sleep, but disturbs and robs you off with other functions and gives you a temporary relief in exchange of much more dangerous consequences.

Consequences that may amount to threat of life and psychological imbalances.

Stress and Depression & AHDH pills (Anxiety Pills)
Stress is the body's reaction to any change that requires an adjustment or response. The body reacts to these changes with physical, mental, and emotional responses.

Stress is a normal part of life. Many events that happens to you and around you—and many things that you do yourself—put stress on your body. You can experience stress from your environment, your body, and your thoughts.

The human body is designed to experience stress and react to it. Stress can be positive, keeping us alert and ready to avoid danger.

Stress becomes negative when a person faces continuous challenges without relief or relaxation between challenges. As a result, the person becomes overworked and stress-related tension builds.

Stress that continues without relief can lead to a condition called distress—a negative stress reaction.

Distress can disturb the body's internal balance or equilibrium, leading to physical symptoms such as headaches, an upset stomach, elevated blood pressure, chest pain, sexual dysfunction, and problems sleeping.

Research suggests that stress also can bring on or worsen certain symptoms or diseases.

Stress also becomes harmful when people use alcohol, tobacco, or drugs to try and relieve their stress.

Unfortunately, instead of relieving the stress and returning the body to a relaxed state, stress pills and other substances tend to keep the body in a stressed state and cause more problems. The distressed person becomes trapped in a vicious circle.

Consider the following:
- Forty-three percent of all adults suffer adverse health effects from stress.
- Seventy-five percent to 90% of all doctor's office visits are for stress-related ailments and complaints.

- Stress can play a part in problems such as headaches, high blood pressure, heart problems, diabetes, skin conditions, asthma, arthritis, depression, and anxiety.
- The Occupational Safety and Health Administration (OSHA) declared stress a hazard of the workplace. Stress costs American industry more than $300 billion annually.
- The lifetime prevalence of an emotional disorder is more than 50%, often due to chronic, untreated stress reactions.

Controlling stress is important to our health. Unrelenting stress can turn to distress. Stress is the body's reaction to any change that requires a physical, mental, or emotional adjustment or response.

Emotional problems can also result from distress. These problems include depression, panic attacks, or other forms of anxiety and worry.

Stress is linked to six of the leading causes of death: heart disease, cancer, lung ailments, accidents, cirrhosis of the liver, and even suicide.

Stress also becomes harmful when people engage in the compulsive use of substances or behaviors to try to relieve their stress.

These substances or behaviors may include food, alcohol, tobacco, drugs, gambling, sex, shopping, and the Internet.

Many medications originally approved for the treatment of stress & depression have been found to relieve symptoms of anxiety.

These include certain selective serotonin reuptake inhibitors (SSRIs), tricyclic antidepressants (TCAs), monoamine oxidase inhibitors (MAOIs), and the newer atypical antidepressants.

Antidepressants are often preferred over the traditional anti-anxiety drugs because the risk for dependency and abuse is smaller.

However, antidepressants take up to 4 to 6 weeks to begin relieving anxiety symptoms, so they can't be taken "as needed."

For example, antidepressants wouldn't help at all if you waited until you were having a panic attack to take them. Their use is limited to chronic anxiety problems that require ongoing treatment.

The antidepressants most widely prescribed for anxiety are SSRIs. These work by regulating serotonin levels in the brain to elevate mood and have been used to treat panic disorder, obsessive-compulsive disorder (OCD), and generalized anxiety disorder (GAD).

Common dangerous effects include:
- Nausea
- Nervousness
- Headaches

- Sleepiness
- Sexual dysfunction
- Dizziness
- Stomach upset
- Weight gain

Although physical dependence is not as quick to develop with antidepressants, eventually **after a long use, it's difficult to escape, withdrawal is certainly a big issue.**

If discontinued too quickly, antidepressant withdrawal can trigger symptoms such as extreme depression and fatigue, irritability, anxiety, flu-like symptoms, and insomnia.

Medication can relieve some symptoms of anxiety, but it also comes with dangerous risks, effects and safety concerns—including the risk of addiction.

Dangers of anti-anxiety drugs
Anti-anxiety drugs work by reducing brain activity. While this temporarily relieves anxiety, it can also lead to unwanted dangerous effects.

The higher the dose, the more pronounced these risks. However, some people feel sleepy, foggy, and uncoordinated even on low doses of benzodiazepines, which can cause problems with work, school, or everyday activities such as driving. Some even feel a medication hangover the next day.

Because anxiety pills are metabolized slowly, the medication can build up in the body when used over longer periods of time.

The result is over sedation. People who are over sedated may look like they're drunk.

Common dangerous effects of anxiety or tranquilizers
- Drowsiness, lack of energy
- Clumsiness, slow reflexes
- Slurred speech
- Confusion and disorientation
- Depression
- Dizziness, lightheadedness
- Impaired thinking and judgment
- Memory loss, forgetfulness
- Nausea, stomach upset
- Blurred or double vision

Anxiety pills are also associated with depression. Long-term pill users are often depressed, and higher doses are believed to increase the risk of both depressive symptoms and suicidal thoughts and feelings.

Furthermore, anxiety drugs can cause emotional blunting or numbness. **The medication relieves the anxiety, but it also blocks feelings of pleasure or pain.**

Paradoxical effects of anti-anxiety drugs : Despite their sedating properties, some people who take anti-anxiety medication experience paradoxical excitement.

The most common paradoxical reactions are increased anxiety, irritability, and agitation. However, more severe effects can also occur, including:

- Mania
- Hostility and rage
- Aggressive or impulsive behavior
- Hallucinations

These adverse effects are dangerous. Paradoxical reactions to these anxiety medications are most common in children, the elderly, pregnant women, people already suffering from stress or depression and people with developmental disabilities.

Remember, stress, depression or any other anxiety medications aren't a cure. Medication may treat some symptoms of anxiety, but can't change the underlying issues and situations in your life that are making you anxious.

Anxiety medication won't solve your problems if you're anxious because of mounting bills, a tendency to jump to "worst-case scenarios", or an unhealthy relationship. That's where therapy and other lifestyle changes come in.

There are many treatment alternatives to medication. Behavior Therapy is widely accepted to be more effective for anxiety than drugs. To overcome anxiety for good, you may also need to make major changes in your life.

Lifestyle changes that can make a difference in anxiety levels include nutritional correction, regular exercise, adequate sleep, and a healthy diet. Other effective treatments for anxiety include talk therapy, meditation, biofeedback, hypnosis, and reflexology.

Recreation Pills
Recreational drug is the use of a drug with the intention of creating or enhancing recreational experience.

Drugs commonly considered capable of recreational use include alcohol, nicotine, caffeine and any other synthetic drugs formulation used for these purpose.

Depressants are used as recreation drugs that temporarily diminish the function or activity of a specific part of the body or mind. Effects may include anxiolysis, sedation, and hypotension.

Due to their effects typically having a "down" syndrome to them, depressants are also occasionally referred to as "downers".

Stimulants or "uppers", which increase mental and/or physical function, are in stark contrast to depressants and are considered to be their functional opposites.

Depressants are widely used throughout the world

When these are used, effects may include anxiolysis, analgesia, sedation, somnolence, cognitive/memory impairment, dissociation, muscle relaxation, lowered blood pressure/heart rate, respiratory depression, anesthesia, and anticonvulsant effects. Some are also capable of inducing feelings of euphoria.

The Pathetic Status of Pill & Pain culture can be summarized as below

- Billions of people around the world are on pills for some reason of the other.
- Billions of people are ready to take any pills thrown unto them by doctors.
- Majority of them do so with the hope of getting cured from their apathy.
- Majority of them are disappointed and have become dependent of these pill on a daily basis.
- Billions of dollars are spent on research and development of pills worldwide yet we do not have a cure for most of the common disorders.

Why ? NOW YOU ALREADY KNOW IT.

CHAPTER 2
HOW WAS IT ALL DISCOVERED

In future people will demand they own their medical records, not the doctor, not the hospital and through technology and education will gain medical freedom. By owning and maintaining their own they will be able to communicate to any medical expert worldwide for wide range of treatment options.

Health is one of the most important aspects of our lives, however, it is also one of the most neglected aspects. we are worried about our education, merits in college, career, salary hike, weather, travelling, increasing fuel rates, and almost everything around us, but seldom do we pay any importance to our health; at least not until we face a problem.

My experience was nothing different than any other human of today's modern world. After years of tiring study of school and colleges, followed by job experience. The world and time passed by and I had no time to think about myself.

Anything else besides success and growth in personal and professional field was non-priority.

Many sleepless nights appeared as enthusiasm and devotion to my work and profession. Obesity, Hypertension and stress were not even noticed because success overpowered the priority in life.

As an Adult, eating out, late night meetings and parties dominated the work week. Family and friends were more important than personal time, health and wellbeing.

I always had a bare minimum palate of food choices, I never took alcohol ever in my life, Never ever tried smoking, by choice never ever bothered for tea, coffee, beverages.

A Complete teetotaler, YET I was obese.

My mother was a Medical Professional. I had practically grown knowing each and every day in a life of a Medical Practitioner.

She was in the Surgery Department all her life and headed the department, most part of her career.

She had a unique habit of sharing all the Details of surgery performed in the operation theatre everyday. The information used to be quite detailed and graphic in nature.

I was always highly interested in her narrations. She did this to remove the stress of the day and maybe that acted as therapy for her.

She spent twenty seven years of her life in one of the largest Government owned hospital in the country.

With all that knowledge and experience of human body she possessed, while working all her live in surgery, surrounded by the world class doctors and other medical practitioners around her, she never had one answer, **why was her kid Obese?**

I was an Obese kid and she didn't have an answer or a solution. With the common fad, fashion and opinion of people around, even the Medical community used to generalize obesity very casually. Maybe they never had the answer.

Everybody used the Standard statements "Too much food and too little physical movement is the cause of obesity".

How simple and how easy to narrate such a complex situation, I though.

My mother knew that the general perception about obesity was not correct. She watched her son being decently disciplined in his eating habits and active.

With only homemade food and a very active physical lifestyle her son was extremely participative in all sports. In fact she had to stop her kid from playing too much, **YET her son was Obese.**

Failing to find any solution, she had no other option than to develop an opinion which would justify the situation.

Her opinion stated, **if you are not sick and troubled then there is no problem.**

This is one of the reasons that though my mother worked in the medical profession, she **NEVER kept any pills** or generic medicine at home.

The idea that "I am not sick, so I do not have to worry" even though I was obese got cemented in my mind and I was never worried. Never gave a single thought about my obesity, because I was rarely sick.

I was a very active and athletic kid. I was considered a very good sports player. I played football (Soccer), Cricket, Hockey and was very active socially since childhood.

I was very popular in all social gathering and was sought after for my involvement, management and coordination of social event in my community.

I was a kind of born events manager. I was least bothered about my obesity. Life continued with all its beauty, when the sudden discomfort popped up.

Life slipped by, years went by, when a sudden bump and a sudden brake made me and my family realize that something was not in order.

I was in my early thirties that my wife took a call to get a basic blood sugar test done. She noticed something was not normal.

The ants in our sparkling clean washroom caught her attention. We both decided to have a blood test. Her test was normal and mine was a whooping 480 mg/dL.

I was shocked as to see my blood sugar results. I questioned myself, how can this happen. I never felt anything strange physically, I was still very active and I was far from feeling sick.

My doctor immediately advised me to change my food habits and prescribed diabetic pills along with insulin injections to control the high blood sugar which was detected.

The doctor I consulted was no stranger. He was a dear friend of mine. He was a diabetologist (Diabetic Specialist) working in a very large and famous Diabetic Clinic in my city. Surprising and Interestingly he was also suffering from Type II Diabetic.

For me this was not a Coincidence.

I grew up, in and around the medical professionals who did not have an answer for my Obesity. Here I am again at this point in my life when I discovered I am Type II diabetic, and I am around an excellent diabetic doctor who himself is suffering from Type II Diabetes and does not have any answer why he can't cure himself.

I was not surprised when he was sympathetic towards me. He was pleased to invite me to the world of daily tablets/pills and insulin shots.

He was trapped for his life. He will have to survive and manage his condition through daily pills all his life. He had no answers, nor any solution for the cure, neither knew how to stop the pills and live a normal life.

His only solution was to take pills or insulin shots and manage his condition throughout his life.

With my knowledge and experience in research, I decided to discover my own study to find the answer for such a disorder and try to find the reason of not having any cure.

Why? I thought should anyone suffer from a condition like diabetes all his life, when someone was not born with such a disorder.

My hypothesis, if something went wrong in the natural process, some imbalance happened, some disorder happened due to certain incorrect choices, then it can also be brought back to order.

The imbalance can be balanced. If it takes years for such disorder to be discovered, then certainly there should be something that can be done to correct it.

After watching myself suffer for about a year I finally hit a breaking point. I couldn't take it any longer.

So, I set out on a journey to discover the solution to my diabetic problem. The same Problems with which you or some of your family members might suffer. Also Millions of other people around the world suffer.

My journey led to my discovery of a very important of the human natural balance system. **The endocrine system**.

The endocrine system is a network of glands that produce and release hormones that help control many important body functions, especially the body's ability to change calories into energy that powers cells and organs.

The endocrine system influences how your heart beats, how your bones and tissues grow, even your ability to make a baby.

It plays a vital role in whether or not you develop diabetes, thyroid disease, growth disorders, sexual dysfunction, and a host of other hormone-related disorders.

Each gland of the endocrine system releases specific hormones into your bloodstream. These hormones travel through your blood to other cells and help control or coordinate many body processes.

Endocrine glands include:
- **Adrenal glands:** Two glands that sit on top of the kidneys that release the hormone cortisol.

- **Hypothalamus:** A part of the lower middle brain that tells the pituitary gland when to release hormones.
- **Ovaries:** The female reproductive organs that release eggs and produce sex hormones.
- **Islet cells in the pancreas:** Cells in the pancreas control the release of the hormones insulin and glucagon.
- **Parathyroid:** Four tiny glands in the neck that play a role in bone development.
- **Pineal gland:** A gland found near the center of the brain that may be linked to sleep patterns.
- **Pituitary gland:** A gland found at the base of brain behind the sinuses. It is often called the "master gland" because it influences many other glands, especially the thyroid. Problems with the pituitary gland can affect bone growth, a woman's menstrual cycles, and the release of breast milk.
- **Testes:** The male reproductive glands that produce sperm and sex hormones.
- **Thymus:** A gland in the upper chest that helps develop the body's immune system early in life.
- **Thyroid:** A butterfly-shaped gland in the front of the neck that controls metabolism.

Major endocrine glands & Few Common Hormonal Disorder Associated Directly or Indirectly with each Imbalance.

1. Pineal gland   : Stress, Depression resulting majority of chronic disorders . . .
2. Pituitary gland : Impaired Growth and Master source of many Disorders . . .
3. Thyroid gland   : Weight Loss, Weight Gain, Metabolic Disorders, Obesity . . .
4. Thymus   : Allergy, Hypersensitivity . . .
5. Adrenal gland   : Libido Loss . . .
6. Pancreas   : Diabetes, Obesity . . .
7. Ovary   : PCOS, Infertility . . .
8. Testes   : Impotence, Infertility . . .

A litter About Pineal Glands: Also known by names such as 'pineal body', 'epiphysis cerebri', 'epiphysis', other than 'third eye', the pineal gland, in ancient times, was associated with great exaggeration of having mystical powers.

The gland produces what is known as melatonin, a hormone, from the amino acid tryptophan. **This hormone, apart from regulating other hormones, maintains the body's circadian rhythm,** which is basically the day/night cycle. This cycle has a critical role to play when falling asleep and waking up.

Have you ever imagined why do we sleep at night or why do we feel sleepy when it is dark? This is because of the pineal gland, which produces more melatonin when it is dark.

Reversely, when we are exposed to bright lights, the melatonin level drops. Any kind of activity which may disrupt this normal cycle can give rise to pineal gland disorders.

Most commonly, any abnormality in the working of the pineal gland, may signify that there is a mishap in the production of melatonin.

For instance, if a person is exposed to too little light during the day or too much light during the night hours, he may be disrupting his pineal gland.

F

Symptoms include, apart from insomnia, increased anxiety, immune suppression, lowered basal body temperature (body temperature in the morning before rising or moving about or eating anything), and an elevated level of estrogen/progesterone ratio.

One more symptom of this disorder is what is known as Seasonal Affective Disorder (SAD). It is defined as a form of depression which is brought upon by the lack or absence of natural light during the winter months.

Treating the disorder of low melatonin production involves minimizing exposure to artificial light after sundown, and promoting a healthy circadian rhythm with the help of exercise and day time light exposure.

Inculcating a fixed schedule for going to bed and waking up helps manage the problem. So also does practicing meditation techniques for reducing stress. For the other disorder, i.e., excess production of melatonin, one must go for regular exposure to light during the day, and avoiding working in night shifts.

Following natural day/night light patterns helps in improving the circadian rhythms of the body and managing stress helps to regulate hormonal production. Not to mention, exercise daily, especially in sunlight.

A litter About Pituitary gland : Pituitary gland is a small pea sized gland situated in the hollow of your nose, behind the nose bridge.

It is attached to the hypothalamus by means of a small, thin stalk. Hypothalamus is situated at the base of the brain and is responsible for controlling the secretion of pituitary gland.

This gland is rightly **called the master gland, since it is responsible for controlling the functions of other glands as well.**

Malfunctioning of the pituitary gland can play havoc in the body as it also controls the secretion of the other glands of the body.

This leads to hormone imbalance in the body. One of the major problems with the pituitary gland is the development of tumors.

Since there are no specific symptoms, most of the problems associated with pituitary gland go undetected for a very long time. They are only detected by accident while diagnosing some other problems.

Human growth hormone deficiency is a condition where the body does not produce enough of growth hormone in the body. This can have different effects on the body depending on the age at which this condition occurs.

• **Oxytocin is a hormone that plays a vital role in childbirth.** It triggers uterine contractions during and after labor, thus encouraging rapid delivery. The same hormone also stimulates the ejection of breast milk, as a response to the sight, sound or suckling of a newborn.

Oxytocin is also known as the "love hormone", for it gets released into the bloodstream during orgasms in both men and women. In men particularly, the hormone helps maintain erections. Recent findings show that, the hormone may be associated with improving emotions such as trust, empathy, and reducing anxiety and stress. In people with autism, a few studies purport that oxytocin may help with social functioning. To add to this, a study conducted at Claremont Graduate University in Claremont, California, showed that, in women, this hormone may boost happiness.

A common disorder of the pituitary gland is the formation of tumors in it. The cells of the gland may malfunction and grow rapidly or may produce small growths and lead to the formation of tumors. Such tumors are, however, not brain tumors and are non-cancerous. These tumors may be of two types; secretory and non-secretory. The former type produces too much hormones, and the latter type keeps the pituitary gland from functioning optimally.

A little about Thyroid gland : Thyroid is one of the largest among the glands that constitute the endocrine system.

The endocrine system regulates various bodily functions like metabolism, growth and sexual development, through the hormones produced by the glands, that form the system. One such gland is the thyroid gland, that is located below the Adam's apple in the neck.

Like other endocrine glands, thyroid too produces hormones that are very important for the bodily reactions.

In order to produce hormones, the thyroid gland needs iodine and tyrosine (amino acid). It is also noted that thyroid cells are the only cells in the human body, that can absorb iodine.

The primary function of the thyroid gland? Of course, it is the production of hormones called T3, T4 and calcitonin. The hormones (T3 and T4) are released directly into the bloodstream, through which, they are transported to every part of the body.

These hormones enter the body cells and control the metabolism that takes place in those cells. In fact, the metabolism that happens in each and every cell is controlled by the thyroid hormones called T3 and T4.

These hormones stimulate the metabolism in the cells, where oxygen and nutrients are converted to energy. As cells work efficiently, it reflects in the functions of the organ too. So, it is also partly responsible for the healthy functioning of the organs like, heart and liver.

Thyroid has an important role in regulating body temperature too. The hormone calcitonin hormone is associated with the regulation of calcium levels in the body.

Any abnormalities of the thyroid gland and the level of hormones produced by it can cause various health problems. The most common thyroid problems are hyperthyroidism, hypothyroidism, goiter and thyroid cancer.

A litter about Thymus : The thymus was known to the ancient Greeks, and its name comes from the Greek word thumos, meaning "anger", or "heart, soul, desire, life", possibly because of its location in the chest, near where emotions are subjectively felt

The thymus is a specialized organ of the immune system. The thymus "educates" T-lymphocytes (T cells), which are critical cells of the adaptive immune system.

One of the most important roles of the thymus is the induction of central tolerance.

The thymus is largest and most active during the neonatal and pre-adolescent periods. By the early teens, the thymus begins to atrophy and thymic stroma is replaced by adipose (fat) tissue. Nevertheless, residual T lymphopoiesis continues throughout adult life.

The type of malfunction falls into one or more of the following major groups: hypersensitivity or allergy, auto-immune disease, or immunodeficiency.

A little about Adrenal Gland : Adrenal glands (also known as suprarenal glands) are endocrine glands that sit at the top of the kidneys. The right adrenal gland is triangular shaped, while the left adrenal gland is semilunar shaped.

The adrenal glands are named for their location relative to the kidneys. The term "adrenal" comes from ad-(Latin, "near") and renes (Latin, "kidney"). "suprarenal" is derived from supra-(Latin, "above") and renes.

They are chiefly responsible for releasing hormones in response to stress through the synthesis of corticosteroids such as cortisol and catecholamines such as epinephrine (adrenaline) and norepinephrine.

Cortisol is the main glucocorticoid under normal conditions and its actions include mobilization of fats, proteins, and carbohydrates, but it does not increase under starvation conditions. Additionally, cortisol enhances the activity of other hormones including glucagon and catecholamines.

The adrenal glands regulate several fundamental aspects of human physiology via secretion of specific hormones including glucocorticoids (eg, cortisol), mineralocorticoids (eg, aldosterone), catecholamines (eg, epinephrine), and adrenal androgens (eg, dehydroepiandrosterone [DHEA])

Glucocorticoids help regulate blood sugar, blood pressure, fat and protein metabolism, and immunity.

Mineralocorticoids help regulate kidney and cardiovascular function (via maintenance of salt and water balance within the body).

Catecholamines help regulate the "fight or flight" response to stress.

Adrenal androgens are precursors to sex hormones such as testosterone and estrogen.

Disordered adrenal function can lead to a barrage of significant complications, including diabetes, high blood pressure, prolonged fatigue, and depression. Addison's disease and Cushing's syndrome are two major adrenal gland disorders, and they can be deadly if left untreated

Adrenal fatigue is a collection of signs and symptoms, known as a syndrome, that results when the adrenal glands function below the necessary level.

Most commonly associated with intense or prolonged stress, it can also arise during or after acute or chronic infections, especially respiratory infections such as influenza, bronchitis or pneumonia.

As the name suggests, its paramount symptom is fatigue that is not relieved by sleep

Adrenal fatigue can wreak havoc with your life. In the more serious cases, the activity of the adrenal glands is so diminished that you may have difficulty getting out of bed for more than a few hours per day.

With each increment of reduction in adrenal function, every organ and system in your body is more profoundly affected. Changes occur in your carbohydrate, protein and fat metabolism, fluid and electrolyte balance, heart and cardiovascular system, and even sex drive.

Many other alterations take place at the biochemical and cellular levels in response to and to compensate for the decrease in adrenal hormones that occurs with adrenal fatigue. Your body does its best to make up for under-functioning adrenal glands, but it does so at a price.

Adrenal fatigue is produced when your adrenal glands cannot adequately meet the demands of stress. The adrenal glands mobilize your body's responses to every kind of stress (whether it's physical, emotional, or psychological) through hormones that regulate energy production and storage, immune function, heart rate, muscle tone, and other processes that enable you to cope with the stress.

Whether you have an emotional crisis such as the death of a loved one, a physical crisis such as major surgery, or any type of severe repeated or constant stress in your life, your adrenals have to respond to the stress and maintain homeostasis. If their response is inadequate, you are likely to experience some degree of adrenal fatigue

Over-stimulation of your adrenals can be caused either by a very intense single stress, or by chronic or repeated stresses that have a cumulative effect

You may be experiencing adrenal fatigue if you regularly notice one or more of the following:
- You feel tired for no reason.
- You have trouble getting up in the morning, even when you go to bed at a reasonable hour.
- You are feeling rundown or overwhelmed.
- You have difficulty bouncing back from stress or illness.
- You crave salty and sweet snacks.
- You feel more awake, alert and energetic after 6PM than you do all day.

A little about Pancreas : The pancreas is a glandular organ in the digestive system and endocrine system of vertebrates. It is both an endocrine gland producing several important hormones, including insulin, glucagon, somatostatin, and pancreatic polypeptide, and a digestive organ, secreting pancreatic juice containing digestive enzymes that assist the absorption of nutrients and the digestion in the small intestine.

These enzymes help to further break down the carbohydrates, proteins, and lipids in the chyme.

The part of the pancreas with endocrine function is made up of approximately a million cell clusters called islets of Langerhans. Four main cell types exist in the islets.

They are relatively difficult to distinguish using standard staining techniques, but they can be classified by their secretion: α cells secrete glucagon (increase glucose in blood), β cells secrete insulin (decrease glucose in blood), delta cells secrete somatostatin (regulates/stops α and β cells) and PP cells, or gamma cells, secrete pancreatic polypeptide.

The islets of Langerhans play an imperative role in glucose metabolism and regulation of blood glucose concentration.

The pancreas as an exocrine gland helps out the digestive system. It secretes pancreatic fluid that contains digestive enzymes that pass to the small intestine. These enzymes help to further break down the carbohydrates, proteins and lipids (fats) in the chyme.

In humans, the secretory activity of the pancreas is regulated directly via the effect of hormones in the blood on the islets of Langerhans and indirectly through the effect of the autonomic nervous system on the blood flow.

Few symptoms of the pancreas disorder :
　　　Pain in the upper abdomen
　　　Loss of appetite
　　　Yellowing of the skin and eyes (jaundice)
　　　Back pain
　　　Bloating
　　　Nausea
　　　Vomiting
　　　Digestive upsets
　　　Passing foul-smelling and fatty faeces.

Some of the disorders that affect the pancreas include:
　　　Acute pancreatitis
　　　Chronic pancreatitis
　　　Pancreatic cancer
　　　Diabetes.

A little about ovaries : The ovaries are a pair of organs that women have. They are located in the pelvis, one on each side of the uterus. Each ovary is about the size and shape of an almond.

The ovaries produce a woman's eggs. If an egg is fertilized by a sperm, a pregnancy can result. Ovaries also make the female hormones estrogen and progesterone. When a woman goes through menopause, her ovaries stop releasing eggs and make far lower levels of hormones.

Problems with the ovaries include
    Ovarian cancer
    Ovarian cysts and polycystic ovary syndrome
    Premature ovarian failure
    Ovarian torsion, a twisting of the ovary

Polycystic ovary syndrome (PCOS) is one of the most common female endocrine disorders. PCOS is a complex, heterogeneous disorder.

PCOS is thought to be one of the leading causes of female subfertility and the most frequent endocrine problem in women of reproductive age.

The principal features are (1) anovulation, resulting in irregular menstruation, amenorrhea, ovulation-related infertility; (2) excessive amounts or effects of androgenic (masculinizing) hormones, resulting in acne and hirsutism; and (3) insulin resistance, often associated with obesity, Type 2 diabetes, and high cholesterol levels.

Finding that the ovaries appear polycystic on ultrasound is common, but not an absolute requirement in all definitions of the disorder. The symptoms and severity of the syndrome vary greatly among affected women.

Common symptoms of PCOS include:
Menstrual disorders: PCOS mostly produces oligomenorrhea (few menstrual periods) or amenorrhea (no menstrual periods), but other types of menstrual disorders may also occur.

Infertility: This generally results directly from chronic anovulation (lack of ovulation).

High levels of masculinizing hormones: The most common signs are acne and hirsutism (male pattern of hair growth), but it may produce hypermenorrhea (very frequent menstrual periods) or other symptoms. Approximately three-quarters of patients with PCOS have evidence of hyperandrogenemia.

Metabolic syndrome: This appears as a tendency towards central obesity and other symptoms associated with insulin resistance. Serum insulin, insulin resistance and homocysteine levels are higher in women with PCOS.

Modern Medical treatment of PCOS is tailored to the patient's goals. Broadly, these may be considered under four categories:
    Lowering of insulin levels
    Restoration of fertility
    Treatment of hirsutism or acne

Restoration of regular menstruation, and prevention of endometrial hyperplasia and endometrial cancer

Women with PCOS are at risk for the following:
Endometrial hyperplasia and endometrial cancer (cancer of the uterine lining) are possible, due to overaccumulation of uterine lining, and also lack of progesterone resulting in prolonged stimulation of uterine cells by estrogen. It is not clear if this risk is directly due to the syndrome or from the associated obesity, hyperinsulinemia, and hyperandrogenism.

Insulin resistance/Type II diabetes. A review published in 2010 concluded that women with PCOS had an elevated prevalence of insulin resistance and type II diabetes, even when controlling for body mass index (BMI). PCOS also makes a woman, particularly if obese, prone to gestational diabetes.
High blood pressure, particularly if obese and/or during pregnancy
Depression/Depression with Anxiety
Dyslipidemia—disorders of lipid metabolism—cholesterol and triglycerides.
Cardiovascular disorder
Strokes
Weight gain
Miscarriage
Sleep apnea, particularly if obesity is present
Non-alcoholic fatty liver disease, again particularly if obesity is present
Acanthosis nigricans (patches of darkened skin under the arms, in the groin area, on the back of the neck)

Autoimmune thyroiditis

In each of these areas, there is considerable debate as to the optimal treatment.

General interventions that help to reduce weight or insulin resistance can be beneficial for all these aims, because they address what is believed to be the underlying cause.

PCOS appears to cause significant emotional distress.

There is not sufficient evidence to conclude an effect from PCOS / PCOS pills have be effective based on a systematic review, **yet billions of women around the world are on pills** to handle this situation.

Is it sensible to take pills? You take your own decision.

The lack of proper nutrition is anyhow considered to be the cause of so many disorders in women around the world.

A woman is always the second in line when it comes to providing proper and balanced nutrition in the family. This attitude of the world and society has evolved into a major imbalance not only in the women's body in general, **but has created a great new epidemic of infertility which is seen so obvious nowadays all around.**

A Little about Testes : Testicles, or testes, make male hormones and sperm. They are two egg-shaped organs inside the scrotum, the loose sac of skin behind the penis. It's easy to injure your testicles because they are not protected by bones or muscles.

The testicles (testis) are part of the male reproductive system. They are located inside the scrotum and make the male hormones. Disorders of the testis can cause sexual dysfunction, infertility and hormonal imbalances.

Testes Disorder Symptoms

Each type of testicular disorder can have different symptoms including swelling or pain in the testicles, painful urination, lumps, sexual dysfunction and the inability to conceive a child.

Treatment for testes disorders depends on the diagnosis. Some conditions such as hydrocele may resolve without treatment. Treatment for other issues such as infertility may require lifestyle changes, hormone treatments.

One function of the testes is to secrete the hormone testosterone. This hormone plays an important role in the development and maintenance of many male physical characteristics. These include muscle mass and strength, fat distribution, bone mass, sperm production, and sex drive.

Erectile dysfunction (the inability to achieve or maintain an erection)
Infertility

Decreased sex drive
Decrease in beard and growth of body hair
Decrease in size or firmness of the testicles
Decrease in muscle mass and increase in body fat
Enlarged male breast tissue
Mental and emotional symptoms similar to those
of menopause in women (hot flashes, mood
swings, irritability, depression, fatigue)

Thus instead of taking various pills for ED or to increase your libido, the males facing such problems may need to think about the root cause of ED.

I have personally known ED making numerous men crazy both socially and personally. The rise in crimes and other societal problems can also be considered as the impact of such serious hormonal problem.

Another important phenomenon is the decrease in the male hormone, creating infertility and reduction of male population who have active male hormones.

The increase in the number of subdued male personality characteristics, are increasingly labeled as a physical deficiency or psychological problems in men and are treated with pills on a regular basis.

In my numerous successful treatments of ED, infertility, decreased sexual desires and sexual function in men throughout my years of practice, I have noticed that The males are too egoistic to discuss their matter of ED or decreased libido.

They would rather prefer to try out every pills available to increase their manhood or their sexuality than discusss the reasons of such cause.

This usually happens with the core concept which is highlighted around the world as manhood and thus the sexual performance or sexual strength becomes the center of male existence according to many.

My suggestion to billions of men around the world is to rethink, when anyone says you lack sexual strength, consider that it is not about the particular part or about the sexual organ only, it is about the complete body.

When your whole body is damaged, imbalanced, due to lack of nutrition and building blocks of human cell, **how can a pill create some strength in only one area of your existence**.

You need and will have to go to the root cause of your problems, hormones are not only for women as is known in popular talks, hormones are also very much responsible for male impotence, ED, reduced or increased libido and all other functions of the human body.

These hormones cannot be treated externally by any pills.

All men around the world will have to realize that if you want your manhood back, you have to go back to the basic of human body building blocks.

Rethink what is the correct nutrition for your body, what is the primal requirement of your body.

Maybe what your body requires is not what you like or have been eating all your life.

Think about this and you may get your answers or at least the direction for our answers.

SO ENDOCRINE DISORDER CAUSED NATURALLY, ACCIDENTLY OR THROUGH IMBALANCE NUTRITION FOR YEARS IS RESPONSIBLE FOR MAJORITY OF YOUR DISORDERS AND PROBLEMS.

The Proper functioning of this endocrine system and the proper management of the various hormones through the endocrine system is the key to so many disorder of human body.

The strength of the endocrine system to manage the hormonal system of the human body, can be provided back to it only through proper and correct natural nutrition.

As the wounded/severed part of your body can be stitched back again, but the healing can only happen with the strength of your body.

No artificial pills or external intervention can give the strength back to the endocrine system. This strength has to evolve natural by your body and the system needs to get balanced, corrected and healed.

So remember before taking any pills, Even the slightest hiccup with the function of one or more of these glands can throw off the delicate balance of hormones in your body and lead to an endocrine disorder.

Causes of Endocrine Disorders
Endocrine disorders are typically grouped into two categories:

Endocrine Disorder that results when a gland produces too much or too little of an endocrine hormone, called a hormone imbalance.

The endocrine's feedback system helps control the balance of hormones in the bloodstream. If your body has too much or too little of a certain hormone, the feedback system signals the proper gland or glands to correct the problem.

A hormone imbalance may occur if this feedback system has trouble keeping the right level of hormones in the bloodstream, or if your body doesn't clear them out of the bloodstream properly.

Types of Endocrine Disorders
There are many different types of endocrine disorders. **Diabetes & Thyroidism, is the most common** endocrine disorder diagnosed in the world.

The symptoms of an endocrine disorder vary widely and depend on the specific gland involved. However, most people with endocrine disorder complain of fatigue and weakness.

Treatment of endocrine disorders through chemical medication is the most complicated, as a change in one hormone level can throw off another.

On the surface the endocrine disorder has specific set of symptoms, however the imbalance in any of the hormones throw the whole balance of the body functions. The complete list of symptoms in case of Endocrine Disorder is provided in the Appendix Section of this book.

The most common problem of the world in the recent few decades is the effect of this imbalance in life of normal people around the world.

The approach of the general public, to handle this imbalance, the strong desire to quick fix the symptoms of such disorders which are not possible has been the reason of this chaos.

This imbalance has caused the gigantic rise in the population of people getting Obese, Depression, Diabetes, Thyroidism, Impotence, Infertility, PCOS, Sleep Disorders, Cholesterol, Chronic Heart Disorders etc

The OBESITY problem has not only been the cause of concern for adults, but has not penetrated to the most important of human species, who are supposed to be the most healthy and who bodies are supposed to be strong enough to protect itself during the growing year. YES our children.

The growing concern is the rise in Child Obesity. Be it the urban or the rural population. Be it rich or poor. More and more population around the world is caught in this un-required Obesity epidemic.

Obesity is just the scratch on the surface, many other disorders like STRESS, Depression, Diabetes, Thyroidism, Impotence, Infertility, PCOS, Sleep Disorders, Cholesterol, Chronic Heart Disorders etc have seen a humongous rise.

The interesting scenario is this large populations which has fallen to these trap are the one who have never give a single thought as to **why they have been the victim** of this hormonal imbalance, rather almost all of them have given the control of their body to quick fix pills which never works to correct their condition.

My understanding of this reason made me explore the various research and hidden information which never comes to public domain. My research made me also search for the cause and the remedy.

My search made me discover the reason for such disorder. Made me understand why such disorder are labeled and promoted as a disease rather than just a condition or disorder which can be made straight or corrected.

My research made me understand the economics of healthcare/sickcare and the business of healthcare/sickcare.

These were so revealing and eye opener for me that I made a decision, never to question the knowledge in the public domain, rather just take own steps to find the real reason for every problem.

This approach to take care of myself rather than finding faults opened doors for personal solutions. I stopped blaming the corporations, the governments, my parents, teachers, the system etc.

I took the approach that self awareness if far more important than Global Awareness.

So I found various ancient Indian literature and various secret information on different human body conditions, which led me to a greater discovery and understanding of the human system.

I no longer believed that Obesity, STRESS, Depression Obesity, Diabetes, Thyroidism, Impotence, Infertility, PCOS, Sleep Disorders, Cholesterol, Chronic Heart Disorders etc. are disease.

I found a way to bring back order into disorder, bring back balance into imbalance, Naturally.

I no longer required pills to take care of my diabetes, I was out of my diabetic condition within nine months, I lost more than thirty percent of my body Fat and body weight.

My Diabetologist Doctor and dear friend was shocked to see my change in body composition, he saw a sleek me and yet did not believe that I no longer take any pills, neither I take any more insulin injections.

For his own satisfaction, he arranged a blood test and was surprised to see that all my results according to his range was normal, yet his medical knowledge and his trust in medicine made him look the other way.

He was not ready to discuss how I did it. He wanted the solution for himself, however his EGO made him do things that ordinarily no friend would do. He chose to ignore my healed condition; my corrected system was not only a challenge to his knowledge, but also for his business and profession.

His life was build around patients who suffer from diabetes, he sold his prescription very convincingly saying even he himself takes it. In such a situation, how could he ever agree to something else?

That was the last day I met my friend, who chose to keep himself away from me. He choose to rather be diabetic and continue taking pills than getting cured. It was obvious why he did that and I respect his choice.

However from that day onwards I focused all my energy and strength to help as many people possible. With due respect and regards to what the doctors or medical professionals feel and believe, I was not in the favor of making any statement against anyone.

I choose to help people who would rather get healed and not blame anyone else for their condition. The blame game has to stop.

We get what we desire, we chose the quick fix solution, we are getting it. We choose the pills, we are getting it.

So stop blaming yourself. Stop blaming anyone else. Stop blaming corporations and governments.

Get back to basics. Take charge of yourself. Take responsibility of your own body. Focus on self awareness rather than Global Awareness. Till then you will have no one else than yourself to judge.

CHAPTER 3
DISORDERS ARE TO BE CORRECTED NOT CONTROLLED OR MANINTANED

Our knowledge is a little island in a great ocean of not known knowledge.
—Isaac Bashevis Singer

Disease—something that takes control and destroys the body is some way. **The Disturbance of EASE = DIS EASE**

A disorder—is an imperfect functioning of part of the body or mind. **The Disturbance of Order = DIS ORDER**

Like many other disorders, Type II Diabetes is a disorder of metabolism. If not brought back into order, continuous state of disorder can lead to various diseases . . .

A disease is an abnormal condition of an organism or part, especially as a consequence of infection, inherent weakness, or environmental stress, that impairs normal physiological functioning.

The terms "disease" and "disorder" are often used interchangeably.

A conversation which too place long time ago, among colleagues made me reflect on the use of these words by general population as well as the medical fraternity and questioned **if there actually is a difference.**

And is the difference significant enough to create a global chaos amongst common population for vested interest.

Disease is lack of Ease : Sickness and the cessation of Normal function. The interruption to operate the way it should.

Dis-order is lack of Order: The body function doesn't cease to operate, the order is displaced. Imbalanced physical or mental condition due to some reason which can be balanced.

Where it gets to be challenging in keeping the distinction straight is that many, if not most long-term disorders left unchecked will lead to some disease or the other.

Unchecked disorders of human body will then certainly lead to systems breakdown. Such is the case, for example, with Alcoholism, which is a disorder.

The addiction starts due to certain psychological issues, which lead to cycles of addiction, when left unchecked, becomes a physiological disease.

In Alcoholics, the physiological component is related to the inability of the body to process alcohol, in a similar way to a diabetic being unable to process sugar.

If you are very ill or chronically ill you must have asked yourself many times: why have these problems chosen me? Will there never be a way to conquer them?

One thing's for sure—disorder or disease, for both the conditions we all share the same goal, which is to prevent it, manage it, treat it and/or find a cure.

Modern medicine has done much in the fields of diseases and emergencies to aid cure.

In most other fields, it is mostly control that it aims for. The thrust, both of clinicians and research **decisively is towards suppression rather than cure.**

What medicine needs to do is propel towards cure on one hand and prevention on the other.

Cure, however, is out of consideration, because it appears unachievable, and prevention is nowhere in the collective consciousness of biomedical researchers and opinion makers, **I suspect probably because it would ultimately make them redundant.**

And the cure and prevention lobby makes only weak noises, if at all, and does not have the clout to change mainstream opinion.

Let me put it a little differently. **What should the modern doctor do?** He should either prevent a disease so it does not occur, or cures it if it does.

What does the modern doctor, do? He neither prevents nor cures in. He only controls and maintains the spread of the disease.

The medical establishment doesn't understand the mechanisms that cause disorders or healing, and because of this they don't know how to cure disorders.

Disorders cannot be cured, it should be healed or corrected.

The current medical system teaches disease management and symptom suppression, which is insufficient to meet our healthcare needs.

A reformed system needs a new paradigm that stresses health promotion and treatments that attempt to correct the underlying causes of disease or to correct the disorder that causes the disease.

Modern medicine has been made into a god by a population of people who look to the doctors and pharmaceutical companies to save them.

The rate of deaths from error at the hands of the medical establishment is equal to destroying six jumbo jets full of people every day!

Consider this is without even taking into account the fact that these figures are lower than actuality, since many errors go unreported or untracked.

And these numbers represent deaths only many others are injured each year due to medical prescription errors.

Modern Medicine doesn't cure anything except, diseases few as noted are . . . tuberculosis, pneumonia, bacterial meningitis, gonorrhea, any bacterial illness you care to name.

Better yet, it can suppress but can't completely prevent many viral and bacterial diseases through vaccination. It's not a coincidence that the human lifespan has increased from 48 years to 77 years in slightly more than a century.

However the period of sickness during this lifespan has also increased. **The delay in death doesn't mean better health; it's only extension of bad health.**

Hormones are named from the Greek word hormon, meaning **"to urge or excite"**, because they were first discovered to play a role in hunger, sex, flight-or-fight response, and many other basic drives. Hormones serve within the body as invaluable messengers, governors of development, and regulators of metabolism.

A hormone is a chemical released by a cell, a gland, or an organ in one part of the body that affects cells in other parts of the organism.

Generally, only a small amount of hormone is required to alter cell metabolism. In essence, it is a chemical messenger that transports a signal from one cell to another.

The hormone binds to the receptor protein, resulting in the activation of a signal transduction mechanism that ultimately leads to cell type-specific responses.

Endocrine hormone molecules are secreted (released) directly into the bloodstream. Their interference with the synthesis, secretion, transport, binding, action, or elimination of natural hormones in the body can change the homeostasis, reproduction, development, and/or behavior of human functions and create imbalance in so many natural functions of the body.

Hormone cells are typically of a specialized cell type, residing within a particular endocrine gland, such as thyroid gland, ovaries, and testes etc.

The hierarchical model normally provided in book and other literature is an oversimplification of the hormonal signaling process.

Cellular recipients of a particular hormonal signal may be one of several cell types that reside within a number of different tissues, as is the case for insulin, which triggers a diverse range of systemic physiological effects.

Different tissue types may also respond differently to the same hormonal signal. Because of this, hormonal signaling is elaborate and very hard to dissect or understand.

Most cells are capable of producing one or more molecules, which act as signaling molecules to other cells, altering their growth, function, or metabolism.

The classical hormones produced by cells are in the endocrine glands and play a major role in the endocrine system to balance the various natural bodily functions.

Hormones have the following effects on the body:
- stimulation or inhibition of growth
- wake-sleep cycle and other circadian rhythms
- mood swings
- induction or suppression of apoptosis (programmed cell death)
- activation or inhibition of the immune system
- regulation of metabolism
- preparation of the body for mating, fighting, fleeing, and other activity
- preparation of the body for a new phase of life, such as puberty, parenting, and menopause
- control of the reproductive cycle
- hunger cravings
- sexual arousal

A hormone may also regulate the production and release of other hormones. Hormone signals control the internal environment of the body through homeostasis.

Hormones are chemical messengers within your body that affect almost all aspects of human function.

Let us introduce ourselves with Few major hormones and their functions.

Ghrelin

Ghrelin is your hunger gremlin. It is produced in your stomach and, like many fat-loss hormones, works with your brain to signal that you are hungry. Reducing calories, in an effort to lose weight, causes an increase in ghrelin.

Even after 12 months of a reduced-calorie diet, research shows that ghrelin levels stay elevated.

In other words, your body never adapts to eating less and constantly sends the "I'm hungry" signal, which is why maintaining weight loss is often harder than losing it in the first place.

Leptin

Leptin is a type of hormone called an adipokine that is released exclusively from fat cells. Leptin interacts with your brain to get your body to eat less and burn more energy.

The more body fat you have, the more leptin your fat cells will release. However, too much body fat leads to too much leptin being released—a condition called leptin resistance. When this occurs, your brain becomes numb to leptin's signal.

To maximize leptin sensitivity, get adequate sleep and pack your diet full of human hormone balancing and strengthening nutrition. Losing weight also enhances leptin sensitivity and gives you some momentum, as the more weight you lose, the more effective leptin will become in your body.

Adiponectin
Adiponectin is another adipokine, but unlike leptin, the leaner your body is the more adiponectin your fat cells will release.

Adiponetin enhances your muscle's ability to use carbohydrates for energy, boosts your metabolism, increase the rate in which your body breaks down fat, and curbs your appetite.

Insulin
Insulin plays a very important role in your body and is key for recovering from exercise, muscle building, and maintaining optimal blood sugar levels.

However, when carbohydrate intakes are high and insulin is left to run wild in the body, it can inhibit the breakdown and burning of stored fat.

Insulin and carbohydrates are very tightly linked. The more carbohydrates you eat, the more insulin will be released.

Glucagon
Glucagon is a hormone that acts directly opposite to insulin. While insulin stores carbohydrates and builds

fat, glucagon is responsible for breaking down stored carbohydrates and fats and releasing them so your body can use them for energy.

CCK

Short for Cholecystokinin, this hormone is released from the cells in your intestines whenever you eat protein or fat.

But CCK doesn't just stay in your gut. Instead, it communicates with your nervous system to flip the satiety switch while simultaneously working with your stomach to slow the rate of digestion.

The end result is that you feel fuller longer. Take full advantage of CCK by making sure you have protein and fat at every meal.

Epinephrine

Known as a fight or flight hormone, epinephrine drives the burning of fat and its release for energy in the body. Epinephrine can also aid in appetite suppression.

Growth Hormone

Considered to be the fountain of youth by many, growth hormone also helps with fat loss. Growth hormone interacts with fat cells and coaxes them to break down and burn stored fat for energy.

Growth hormones Stimulates protein synthesis (muscle tone/development), and strength of bones, tendons, ligaments, and cartilage.

Growth Hormones Decreases use of glucose and increases use of fat as a fuel during exercise. This helps to reduce body fat and to keep blood glucose at a normal level.

Endorphins
An endogenous opioid from the pituitary gland that blocks pain, decreases appetite, creates a feeling of euphoria (the exercise high), and reduces tension and anxiety.

Testosterone
An important hormone in both males and females for maintaining muscle tone/volume/strength, increasing basal metabolic rate (metabolism), decreasing body fat, and feeling self-confident. It's produced by the ovaries in females and by the testes in males.

Testosterones in Females have only about one tenth the amount of testosterone that males do, but even at that level in females it also plays a role in libido and intensity of orgasms.

Production of testosterone in females begins to decline as a woman begins to approach menopause (usually late thirties) and in males it begins to decline in his forties.

Estrogen
The most biologically active estrogen, 17 beta estradiol, increases fat breakdown from body fat stores so that it can be used and fuel, increases basal

metabolic rate (metabolism), elevates your mood, and increases libido.

This hormone is at much higher blood levels in females, but the ovaries begin to produce less of it as a woman begins to approach menopause.

Thyroxine (T4)
A hormone produced by the thyroid gland, Thyroxine raises the metabolic rate ("metabolism") of almost all cells in the body. This increase in "metabolism" helps you to feel more energetic and also causes you to expend more energy, and thus is important in weight loss and bringing back balance in other disorders.

6. Epinephrine
A hormone produced primarily by the adrenal medulla that increases the amount of blood the heart pumps and directs blood flow to where it's needed.

Epinephrine Stimulates breakdown of glycogen (stored carbohydrate) in the active muscles and liver to use as fuel. It also stimulates the breakdown of fat (in stored fat and in active muscles) to use as fuel.

Glucagon
A hormone that is also secreted by the pancreas, but it's job is to raise blood levels of glucose ("blood sugar"). When blood sugar levels get too low, glucagon is secreted and causes stored carbohydrate (glycogen) in the liver to be released into the blood stream to raise blood sugar to a normal level. It also

causes the breakdown of fat so that it can be used as fuel.

So, next time you're suffering from any disorder, think about what's might have gone imbalance in the all the wonderful hormonal systems.

The things that are happening to your hormones might even make you want to stop popping pills and focus on taking steps to balance back to this wonderful system

When we differentiated between Disorder and Disease, I primarily explained why it is important to separate the two.

To understand if we require immediate emergency assistance or proper detailed discovery of the root cause to correct or balance the root cause.

The conditions cause by external or alien organism within the human system to cause imminent danger to the survival of one or more human should be termed as disease and should be given immediate medical attention to bring survival chances to any human.

Sometimes to save lives of one or many, it becomes more important to suppress the symptoms than to find the cause or treat the cause.

The priority to provide surviving opportunity to an individual supersedes any other results of the medication. Which no one in the world would object?

Survival is of prime importance in such imminent life threatening situations.

However once out of immediate threat to life, the continued effort by an individual or the medical practitioner to find the root cause and eliminate the root cause is hardly given significance.

Every disorder if not corrected for a very long time or if left unchecked or unbalance will eventually become a disease.

So the understanding to safeguard your basic natural systems is very essential and useful ins protecting us from disorders of natural cause.

Let us explore few of the very common and major disorder around the world. What is the standard story and what might be the actual reasons of such Disorders

OBESITY & Overweight is a Disorder
The causes of obesity or overweight is the result of so many factor. At the core obesity or overweight is a symptom of many different type of disorders. The need today is to understand the reason why someone is overweight or obese.

The Standard Story
You overeat and do not move much so your are fat, overweight or obese.

So if you eat less and move more you can reduce your weight and fat from your body.

Wow !!! What a simplification

Many of you, I wonder, have fallen victim at one time or other to this unfounded theory of balancing calories? You will certainly have come across obese people who were actually starving themselves to death.

This is especially common among women. Psychiatrists' consulting-rooms are full of women being treated for depression induced by trying to follow such a diet.

They have become dependent on this vicious circle, knowing that breaking away from it will only entail putting back on more weight than they have lost.

What actually happens : The hormone story.
Obesity is caused by a hormonal phenomenon, specifically by the consumption of refined carbohydrates, starches and sugars, all of which prompt sooner or later excessive insulin secretion.

Insulin is the primary regulator of fat storage. When insulin levels are elevated, fat accumulates in our body tissue; when they fall, fat is released and we use it for fuel.

By stimulating insulin secretion, carbohydrates make us fat; by driving us to accumulate fat, they increase hunger and decrease the energy we expend in metabolism and physical activity.

In short, obesity is caused not by overeating or sedentary behavior, but by hormonal malfunctioning triggered by the consumption of particular types of carbohydrate containing foods.

The hormones leptin, insulin, oestrogens, androgens and growth hormone influence our appetite, metabolism and body fat distribution.

People who are obese have hormone levels that encourage the accumulation of body fat.

If you haven't been successful in the past, chances are, one or more the following hormonal imbalances could your culprit

Inflammation
Digestive disorders, allergies, autoimmune disease, arthritis, asthma, eczema, acne, abdominal fat, headaches, depression or sinus disorders are associated with chronic inflammation, which has become recognized as the root cause of obesity

Insulin excess
Insulin is an essential substance whose main function is to process sugar in the bloodstream and carry it into cells to be used as fuel or stored as fat.

There are several reasons for excess insulin, but the main culprits are: stress, consuming too many nutrient-poor carbohydrates (the type found in processed foods, sugary drinks and sodas, packaged low-fat foods and artificial sweeteners), insufficient protein intake, inadequate fat intake and deficient fibre consumption.

Unfortunately our body typically responds to these unpleasant feelings by making us think we're hungry, which causes us to reach for high-sugar foods and drinks. We then end up in a vicious cycle of hormonal imbalance, a condition called insulin resistance or metabolic syndrome which only furthers weight gain and our risk of diabetes and heart disease.

Depression or anxiety
Serotonin exerts a powerful influence over our mood, emotions, memory, cravings (especially for carbohydrates), self-esteem, pain tolerance, sleep habits, appetite, digestion and body temperature regulation. When we're depressed or down, we naturally crave more sugars and starches to stimulate the production of serotonin.

When we measure our current lifestyle against all the elements necessary for the body's natural production of serotonin, the wide ranging epidemic of low serotonin is certainly not surprising. Add in chronic stress and multitasking—two of the main causes of serotonin depletion—and it's a wonder any one of us has been left unaffected by low serotonin.

Chronic stress

Under situations of chronic stress—whether the stress is physical, emotional, mental or environmental, real or imagined—our bodies release high amounts of the hormone cortisol.

If you have a mood disorder like anxiety, depression, posttraumatic stress disorder or exhaustion, or if you have a digestive issue such as irritable bowel syndrome, you can bet your body is cranking up your cortisol.

Through a complicated network of hormonal interactions, prolonged stress results in a raging appetite, metabolic decline, belly fat and a loss of hard-won, metabolically active muscle tissue. In other words, stress makes us soft, flabby and much older than we truly are

Toxic estrogen

Excess estrogen in both sexes to be as great a risk factor for obesity as poor eating habits.

There are two ways to accumulate excess estrogen in the body: we either produce too much of it on our own or acquire it from our environment or diet.

We're constantly exposed to estrogen-like compounds in foods that contain toxic pesticides, herbicides and unnatural/chemical based growth hormones.

A premenopausal woman with estrogen dominance will likely have PMS, too much body fat around the hips and difficulty losing weight.

Menopausal women and men may experience low libido, memory loss, poor motivation, depression, loss of muscle mass and increased belly fat.

Low testosterone
Testosterone enhances libido, bone density, muscle mass, strength, motivation, memory, fat burning and skin tone in both men and women. When testosterone is low, an increase of body fat and loss of muscle may still happen—even with dieting and exercise.

Testosterone levels tend to taper off with age, increased obesity and stress, but today men are experiencing testosterone decline much earlier in life—an alarming finding, considering low testosterone has been linked to depression, obesity, osteoporosis, heart disease and even death.

Many researchers blames the proliferation of endocrine-suppressing, estrogen-like compounds used in pesticides and other farming chemicals for the downward trend in male testosterone levels. Phthalates, commonly found in cosmetics, soaps and most plastics are another known cause of testosterone suppression.

Hypothyroidism
Without enough thyroid hormone, every system in the body slows down. Those who suffer from hypothyroidism feel tired, tend to sleep a lot, experience constipation and weight gain typically occurs.

Extremely dry skin, hair loss, slower mental processes, feeling cold, brittle hair, splitting nails, diminished ability to sweat during exercise, infertility, poor memory, depression, decreased libido and an inability to lose weight are also symptoms to watch for.

If you suspect you have a thyroid condition, make sure you assesses your full range of symptoms, not just your blood work.

Even levels of TSH (an indicator of thyroid function) within the normal range has been proven to accelerate weight gain and to interfere with a healthy metabolic rate in both men and women.

These are few or the prominent reason, besides there are can be other reasons that may be contributing to the accumulation of fat in your cells like lipophilia.

Diabetes is a Disorder
Diabetes is a disorder characterized by hyperglycemia or elevated blood glucose (blood sugar). Our bodies function best at a certain level of sugar in the bloodstream.

If the amount of sugar in our blood runs too high or too low, then we typically feel bad. Diabetes is the name of the condition where the blood sugar level consistently runs too high. Diabetes is the most common endocrine disorder.
The three main types of diabetes are
- type 1 diabetes
- type 2 diabetes

- gestational diabetes

Type 1 Diabetes

Type 1 diabetes is an autoimmune disease. An autoimmune disease results when the body's system for fighting infection—the immune system—turns against a part of the body.

In diabetes, the immune system attacks and destroys the insulin-producing beta cells in the pancreas. The pancreas then produces little or no insulin. A person who has type 1 diabetes must take insulin daily to live.

At present, scientists do not know exactly what causes the body's immune system to attack the beta cells, but they believe that autoimmune, genetic, and environmental factors, possibly viruses, are involved.

Type 1 diabetes accounts for about 2 to 5 percent of diagnosed diabetes in the world It develops most often in children and young adults but can appear at any age.

Type 2 Diabetes

The most common form of diabetes is type 2 diabetes. About 95 to 98 percent of people with diabetes have type 2.

This form of diabetes is most often associated with older age, obesity, family history of diabetes, previous history of gestational diabetes, physical inactivity, and certain ethnicities.

About 80 percent of people with type 2 diabetes are overweight or obese.

Type 2 diabetes is increasingly being diagnosed in children and adolescents.

When type 2 diabetes is diagnosed, the pancreas is usually producing enough insulin, but for unknown reasons the body cannot use the insulin effectively, a condition called insulin resistance. After several years, insulin production decreases.

The result is the same as for type 1 diabetes—glucose builds up in the blood and the body cannot make efficient use of its main source of fuel.

The symptoms of type 2 diabetes develop gradually. Their onset is not as sudden as in type 1 diabetes. Symptoms may include fatigue, frequent urination, increased thirst and hunger, weight loss, blurred vision, and slow healing of wounds or sores. Some people have no symptoms.

Gestational Diabetes

Some women develop gestational diabetes late in pregnancy. Although this form of diabetes usually disappears after the birth of the baby, women who have had gestational diabetes have a 40 to 60 percent chance of developing type 2 diabetes within 5 to 10 years.

Maintaining a reasonable body weight and being physically active may help prevent development of type 2 diabetes.

About 3 to 8 percent of pregnant women in the United States develop gestational diabetes. As with type 2 diabetes, gestational diabetes occurs more often in some ethnic groups and among women with a family history of diabetes.

Gestational diabetes is caused by the hormones of pregnancy or a shortage of insulin. Women with gestational diabetes may not experience any symptoms.

Standard Story of Diabetes

Diabetes is a disorder of metabolism—the way the **body uses digested food for growth and energy**. Most of the food people eat is broken down into glucose, the form of sugar in the blood. Glucose is the main source of fuel for the body.

After digestion, glucose passes into the bloodstream, where it is used by cells for growth and energy. **For glucose to get into cells, insulin must be present. Insulin is a hormone** produced by the pancreas, a large gland behind the stomach.

When people eat, the pancreas automatically produces the right amount of insulin to move glucose from blood into the cells.

In people with diabetes, however, the pancreas either **produces little or no insulin,** or the cells do not respond appropriately to the insulin that is produced. Glucose builds up in the blood, overflows into the urine, and passes out of the body in the urine. **Thus,** the body loses its main source of fuel even though the blood contains large amounts of glucose.

What Actually happens : The Hormone Story
Diabetes is a very complex issue. It starts as a metabolic syndrome that is a combination of nutritional and hormonal imbalances. It's important to correct these imbalances

Diabetes actually is, in a sense, a consequence of hormonal imbalance. It all starts with imbalances in the hormone insulin that lead to glucose intolerance

All of your hormones work together and affect each other, so imbalances of other hormones can lead to insulin imbalances or insulin resistance.

All of your hormones work together and affect each other, so imbalances of other hormones can lead to insulin imbalances or insulin resistance. This may be particularly evident around menopause.

During perimenopause, your progesterone levels decline. This decline in progesterone affects your insulin metabolism and, as your progesterone levels become low, you develop a predisposition to glucose intolerance.

High levels of cortisol, which is produced by your adrenal glands in response to stress, can also lead to glucose intolerance.

In fact, this can lead to an unhealthy cycle, because diabetes can affect your adrenals, causing them to produce more cortisol, which in turn can make your diabetes worse.

Diabetes is sometimes a feature of a more complex endocrine syndrome than the deficiency of insulin, the disorder is partly caused by excess of various hormones.

Insulin
Insulin is produced by the islets of Langerhans in the pancreas. It leads to diabetes, when it is not produced in sufficient quantities, or when it is used inefficiently by the body.

During the process of digestion, food is converted into glucose that is sent to the bloodstream.

Additionally, glucose provides the cells with energy, so that they can carry out their designated functions.

Normally, insulin moves glucose from the bloodstream to cells, but with diabetes, high amounts of glucose remain in the bloodstream as a result of issues with insulin.

Cortisol
Cortisol is a hormone produced by the adrenal glands. Its production is regulated by another hormone called corticotropin, or ACTH.

The pituitary gland in the brain produces ACTH and when it is released into the bloodstream, it stimulates the adrenal glands to produce cortisol.

Some of the functions of cortisol include regulating blood pressure, helping the body cope with stress such as surgery or illness, and regulating glucose production.

Excessive quantities of cortisol in the body can lead to diabetes because it inhibits the effects of insulin and stimulates the liver to produce glucose. Cushing's syndrome is a condition that occurs when the adrenal glands produce too much cortisol.

Growth Hormone
The pituitary gland produces many hormones including growth hormone. Functions of growth hormone include growth and development of muscles, bones and other organs in the body.

Overproduction of this hormone in adults causes a disease called acromegaly. Acromegaly is characterized by thickening and deformation of the bones. Diabetes can be a consequence of acromegaly.

The excess in growth hormone that occurs in acromegaly increases blood glucose levels by inhibiting movement of glucose into the cells, and this may then lead to diabetes.

All hormones are interdependent, thus such imbalance in the above mentioned hormones can also be caused by disruption or disturbance in other hormones that regulate the endrocrine system. So the major causes cannot be project sas the only cause, the full picture needs to be seen. Thus Diabetes is a disorder which if required to be cured needs to be corrected. No amount of medicines or pills will be useful if this balance is not based on natural balancing of the hormones. The building blocks of such a complex system depends on the nutrition body depends on. Focus and you will be out of such conditions like diabetes.

Thyroidism is a Disorder
The thyroid gland is a butterfly-shaped organ located in the front of the neck, just over the windpipe. It produces iodine-containing hormones which regulate the rate at which body cells use energy and produce heat.

The growth and development of all the body's tissues are dependent on the thyroid gland's proper functioning. If the thyroid gland is either overactive or underactive, it can create health problems.

Standard Story of Thyroidism
A person with too little secretion of thyroid hormone, called hypothyroidism, has general symptoms of slowing down—coldness, sluggishness, dry skin and scanty hair growth. In more serious cases, there is a characteristic thickening of the skin, a condition called myxedema.

At the opposite extreme, the person with an overactive thyroid gland, called hyperthyroidism, may have an increase in body metabolism, which results in weight loss in spite of an increased appetite, excessive warmth and sweating, noticeably trembling hands, pounding of the heart and, in some cases, bulging eyes.

Along with these symptoms, the thyroid gland may swell. This swelling is called a goiter.

What actually happens : The Hormone Story
Thyroid hormone (TH)
TH is produced by the thyroid, a butterfly-shaped gland behind the larynx, in response to thyroid stimulating hormone (TSH), which is released by the pituitary gland.

TH exists in two major forms. Levothyroxine (T4), with four iodine atoms per molecule, is an inactive form that can be converted into T3, and is produced exclusively by the thyroid gland. Triiodothyronine (T3), with three iodine atoms per molecule, is eight times more effective than T4. It is converted from T4 in the thyroid, brain, liver, and bloodstream, and in various tissues of the body.

The Role of TH in the Body : One important function of TH is helping the body convert food into energy and heat. T3 directly boosts energy metabolism in mitochondria, the powerhouses of cells.

T3 triggers rapid protein synthesis and influences mitochondrial gene transcription, the reading of genes and synthesis of proteins from genetic information. These activities cause breakdown of proteins and an increase in free fatty acids, as well as increased oxygen use. TH elevates the heart rate to meet the increased oxygen needs.

TH also regulates body temperature. TSH, which stimulates the thyroid to produce TH, also stimulates brown adipose tissue, a mitochondria-rich tissue, to boost heat production in mammals without muscle activity.

TH fluctuates in response to energy intake and external temperature. During starvation, the body naturally lowers TH, not only to reduce energy needs, but also to prevent ketone bodies from building up in the blood and kidneys.

Ketone build-up, which can also happen in diabetes, can cause damage to the kidneys and other part of the body. Injury and illness lower TH levels, which rebound once the patient is healed.

TH is very sensitive to the levels of other hormones besides TSH. Estrogen partially blocks the efficiency of TH, so women compensate by producing more TH than men.

This may be why women have larger thyroids than men and are more prone to thyroid disease of all types. Women who take TH replacement pills increase their TH dosage when they start taking birth control pills, to compensate for the higher levels of estrogen from birth control pills. Growth hormone also partially blocks TH, but it also complements TH in its effects on growth, development, and metabolism.

We still do not know all the genes that are regulated by TH.

This allows many different genes to come under the control of TH without the genes themselves mutating. Different species may have different genes under control of TH, especially these concerned with development.

Most chemicals that cause hypothyroidism do not block thyroid receptors in the genes; they only block the efficiency or synthesis of TH.

Hence most of our information about which genes are regulated by TH comes from studying genetic disorders in which the TRs are non-functional.

Clinical effects are less severe than with congenital hypothyroidism and can include short stature, delayed bone maturation, hyperactivity, learning disabilities, and hearing defects, as well as mixed features of hyper—and hypothyroidism. This condition is usually inherited dominantly.

Pendred's Syndrome is caused by a defect that limits the incorporation of iodine into thyroid hormone, which wrecks the structure of the hormone.

People who develop hypothyroidism later in life may have ringing in their ears and dulled hearing.

TSH has unknown effects on lymphocytes and brain cells; therefore imbalances affecting TSH levels may cause additional, unknown effects on the brain and immune system. One mutation was found in association with Graves' disease.

Graves' disease is an autoimmune form of hyperthyroidism, and the genes that seem to increase risk of Graves' disease are associated with immunity.

In humans, thyroid hormone plays a notable role in brain development from the middle of pregnancy to the second year of life.

Maternal or fetal hypothyroidism, whether caused by lack of iodine during the pregnancy, or by other problems, can cause a non-genetic condition called cretinism.

Babies affected by cretinism can develop normal intelligence if the condition is remedied within a few months, but otherwise they suffer severe, irreversible mental retardation.

Effects of TH Imbalance: Hypothyroidism
Some of the most profound effects of TH imbalance are in the mental arena. Hypothyroid people sleep easily and do not get full refreshment from their sleep.

During waking hours, they experience fatigue, apathy, and "brain fog" (short-term memory problems and attention deficits). These problems may affect their daily functioning and cause increased stress and depression.

TH acts as a neurotransmitter. TH imbalance can mimic psychiatric disease because T3 influences levels of serotonin, a neurotransmitter integral to moods and behavior. Low levels of T3 can cause depression.

Some anti-depressants make hypothyroid patients feel even worse because the medications depress T3 levels.

Paradoxically, some substances labelled depressants such as alcohol or opiates can increase T3 levels by impairing the breakdown of T3 in the brain, thus lifting mood. This may be one reason why these substances are so addictive.

Severe hypothyroidism can cause symptoms similar to Alzheimer's disease: memory loss, confusion, slowness, paranoid depression, and in extreme stages, hallucinations.

Thyroid disorder is one of the many treatable disorder that must be ruled out before arriving at the diagnosis.

Risk of hypothyroidism increases with age; by age 60, 17% of women and 9% of men have symptoms of thyroid disorder.

Low TH levels also produce fatigue, slight hypoglycemia (low blood sugar), slowed digestion of food, and constipation. Infertility is common.

These symptoms can indicate that other disorder are present, particularly because TH levels tend to go down during prolonged illness in an effort to conserve energy. Chronic disease, such as Lyme disease, can mimic (or cause) hypothyroidism.

Hypothyroidism is not difficult to diagnose by symptoms, if the patient reports enough symptoms to the doctor and if the doctor thinks of it. **Diagnosis can be confirmed by blood tests, but the cause is less easy to discern.**

TH imbalance has a profound effect on cardiovascular fitness because TH helps control heart rate and blood pressure. Under hypothyroid conditions, the heart can slow to 30 heart beats a minute and develop arrhythmia. Blood pressure may fall from normal levels of 120/90 to 70/50.

Hypothyroidism also weakens muscles, including the diaphragm. As a result, breathing can become less efficient. A goiter impairs breathing even more. Snoring may start or become worse.

Fatigue sets in easily; in fact it never quite leaves a person with symptomatic hypothyroidism. Muscles and joints often ache. With respiration impaired and oxygen in short supply, exercise takes a heavy toll on the body, and muscles do not strengthen in response to exercise; nor does stamina improve.

Low thyroid levels actually trigger muscle fibers to change their type, from fast-twitch fibers to slow-twitch fibers. This may be an adaptive strategy for coping with starvation, since blood sugar is low under hypothyroid conditions and fast-twitch muscle fibers require high levels of glucose to operate.

Fatty acid levels in the blood are elevated to provide fuel for the fat-burning slow-twitch muscles. However, low oxygen in the blood due to slow heart rate and respiratory problems limits the slow-twitch muscles' effectiveness.

Even after receiving treatment for hypothyroidism, many people find that their energy needs and ability to handle physical labor have changed permanently.

Strength training can help restore their fitness, but only after thyroid hormone levels have normalized naturally.

Hypothyroidism is the second leading cause of high cholesterol, after diet. When TH levels drop, the liver no longer functions properly and produces excess cholesterol, fatty acids, and triglycerides, which increase the risk of heart disease. High cholesterol may also contribute to the risk of Alzheimer's disease.

Iodine overdose rarely is a problem, as the thyroid gland stores iodine until it is necessary, and releases TH in the less active T4 form, and TH is also bound up by transport proteins in the blood until it is needed.

Some experts believe that continual iodine overdoses leads to autoimmune thyroid disease, because it seems to be the major cause of thyroid disorder in developed countries.

Two autoimmune thyroid diseases, Graves' disease and Hashimoto's thyroiditis, are thought to be inherited, but have not been linked positively to any genes.

Autoimmune thyroid disease is identified by detecting antibodies in the blood. In the case of Graves' disease, antibodies latch onto an enzyme essential for making T4, and keep it active and continually turned on.

Some experts have suggested that autoimmune thyroid disorder develops as a result of iodine overconsumption. Both the U.S. and Japan have high levels of iodine consumption and of autoimmune thyroid disease.

Japanese people consume iodine because seafood makes up a large proportion of the diet, and Americans do because salt is iodinated and the food industry uses iodine as a machine wash.

Other experts believe that pollutants are a more important factor. Pollutant chemicals like polychlorinated biphenyls (PCBs) and dioxins have been shown to interfere with thyroid function and are more prevalent in industrialized countries where thyroid disease levels are high.

Autoimmune thyroid disease, either hyperthyroidism or hypothyroidism, is also linked to post-traumatic stress disorder and is often first observed clinically after periods of prolonged stress.

Other studies are uncovering the role of TH in the brain, and finding new causes of thyroid hormone metabolism disorders.

Such research provides hope that autoimmune thyroid disease can one day be attacked at its source.

However, adequate information has not spread into the medical field. Labs performing blood work use overly broad normal ranges of TSH levels.

Thyroid disease affects 8 times as many women as men, possibly because women need higher levels of TH than men do, but it has no age, gender, or ethnic barriers.

Patients may have some or all the obvious symptoms: fatigue, lack of focus, depression, constipation, anxiety attacks, dry hair, dry skin, edema (swelling), lack of exercise tolerance, weight gain (especially in the stomach), muscle and joint pains, problems swallowing (due to enlarged thyroid), goiter, facial puffiness, unusual new headaches, loss of eyebrows, lack of sex drive, lowered body temperature, low or high blood pressure, and slowed heart rate.

The link between high cholesterol and underlying hypothyroidism is vastly overlooked.

People have their cholesterol tested more regularly than their thyroid hormone levels. The result is prescriptions for expensive cholesterol-lowering drugs that don't address the real problem.

People diagnosed with high cholesterol, especially those with low body temperature, should have their thyroid function tested before they begin taking such drugs.

Also, smokers and other substance abusers should be watched for hypothyroidism (and urged to quit), as stimulants and depressants both can affect TH metabolism.

Researchers need to understand the proper function of thyroid hormone and the pathology of thyroid disorder to fully understand how our bodies, brains, and immune systems develop and work, in health and in illness.

It is impossible to know the prevalence of thyroid disorder and figure out all the causes if patients take years on average to be diagnosed.

We still do not know what causes the high prevalence of autoimmune thyroid disorder in developed countries.

Similarly **Impotence is a Disorder, Infertility is a Disorder, PCOS is a Disorder, Sleep Disorders is a Disorder, Imbalanced Cholesterol is disorder, Chronic Heart Disorders is a Disorder, STRESS & Depression**

is a Disorder and almost all of these and many more disorder are due the imbalance caused in the hormone system of human body.

Should you not reconsider balancing this imbalances which has been and is causing so many disorders, rather than jumping into the bandwagon of popping popular pills, and creating much larger chaos in your system than it might naturally cause.

Make informed decision; think about hormone first if the cause of disorder has evolved naturally. And the answers to these disorder might be very much in the natural balancing of your human hormone system.

Why modern medical science still do not have answer for cancer, although Ancient Indian healing and Cure never even considered cancer different from any other disorder

Many cancers are hormonal related. Estrogen dominance may be accountable for breast, prostate, cervix, endometrial, uterine, and ovarian cancer, for example.

Many researchers attribute the high incidence of these cancers to the ubiquitous presence of environmental estrogen (also called xenobiotics) that is present in our food such as commercially raised poultry and cattle; pesticides; and common household goods such as plastics that contain estrogen like compounds.

Phyto-estrogens such as soy and DIM are natural weak estrogen from food that is has 1/500 the potency of estrogen in our body.

They work by competitively inhibiting the estrogen receptor site on the cell membrane, thereby preventing estrogen from exerting its effect on the cell.

These phytoestrogen also exert a weak estrogen effect by themselves and therefore intake should be monitored to avoid excessive estrogen in the body. Hormone replacement must be taken with care since some cancers are hormone sensitive.

Maintaining hormonal balance is a key factor in preventing cancer and reversing hormone sensitive cancers.

Cancers such as breast and prostate cancer are closely linked to estrogen dominance syndrome.

Normalization of estrogen in our body can be achieved naturally.

Thus I let you decide if the popular course of action in cancer cure or treatment is really the best one.

Or should our general populations start taking their own body and health decision based on informed knowledge and alternate perspective.

Tackle, handle, manage, treat or cure cancer with a different perspective rather than the popular pills culture dominated path which anyhow eventually leads to painful death or pills dependent suffering life.

Give life a chance, rather than subjecting it to cuts, radiation and burn that would never heal, rather take the power to heal your life out of your body.

Help yourself and your loved one to, not get emotionally involved with the modern medical advancement which still does not have a cure, rather everything else than cure.

CHAPTER 4
IMBALANCE CANNOT BE CURED, BUT IT CAN BE BALANCED

Let me tell you something you already know. The world ain't all sunshine and rainbows. It is a very mean and nasty place It will beat you to your knees and keep you there permanently if you let it. You, me or nobody is going to hit as hard as life. But it ain't about how hard you're hit, it is about how hard you can get hit and keep moving forward, how much can you take and keep moving forward. That's how winning is done!

—Rocky Balbo
—A fictional Character in the Movie Rocky

OBESITY & Overweight is an Imbalance
Diabetes is an Imbalance
Thyroidism is an Imbalance
Impotence is an Imbalance
Infertility is an Imbalance
PCOS is an Imbalance
Sleep Disorders is an Imbalance
Cholesterol is disorder is an Imbalance
Chronic Heart Disorders is an Imbalance

STRESS & Depression is an Imbalance Cancer is an imbalance . . . .

Should I say more, all the above mentioned and many more not mentioned disorders which occur naturally due to constant degradation of the human cell.

All these occur due to constant degeneration of human body and the strength of the human natural system.

When anyone want to tackle any of these and other disorders immediately and does not realize that to even improve the situation through quick fix you would first need to give the strength to the human core system to hold it together again.

If you go for any sort of medication for any disorder, it is vitally important that you first understand the need of nourishing the human body and human system naturally.

Unless one understand this, all steps towards curing any disorder or disease would be futile.

Natural **Nutrition** that is needed and required by your body needs to be studied by allmost majority of the population of the world. Such basic need is not known to majority of us. The basic bio-chemistry is not known and we pop pill as if we are the scholar of the chemical industry.

I have known and seen people discussing chemicals and pharmacy as if their were Nobel Laureates and

Professors of chemical engineering, and when asked about their own body's organic chemistry or their daily food organic chemistry, they become dumb or talk like dumbs.

Thus ignorance, illiteracy and arrogance on this basic information about our body and food, has made us the victim of such huge disorder and chaos.

It's time for all of us to take a step back, refocus, realign, rethink, if it is worth to throw our beautiful life and such miraculous human body system to some quick fix pills and medication.

Should we not give this amazing creation called human body system a chance, an opportunity to live a disorder FREE, pills FREE, medication FREE and imbalance FREE LIFE

You can start with this basic knowledge to understand the basic biochemistry of human body and the food which is required to maintain this basic biochemistry

Proteins
Proteins compose over 50% of the dry weight of an average living cell and are very complex macromolecules. They also play a fundamental role in the structure and function of human cells.

Consisting mainly of carbon, nitrogen, hydrogen, oxygen, and some sulfur, they also may contain iron, copper, phosphorus, or zinc.

In humans, proteins are essential for growth and survival, they are the building blocks of each cell in the human system and vary depending upon a person's age and physiology (e.g., pregnancy). Proteins greather than 50% of the food item for humans are commonly found is in Nuts, Meat, poultry, and seafood.

Proteins are large biological molecules consisting of one or more chains of amino acids.

Proteins perform a vast array of functions within living organisms, including catalyzing metabolic reactions, replicating DNA, responding to stimuli, and transporting molecules from one location to another.

Proteins differ from one another primarily in their sequence of amino acids

Like other biological macromolecules, proteins are essential parts of organisms and participate in virtually every process within cells.

Many proteins are enzymes that catalyze biochemical reactions and are vital to metabolism.

The chief characteristic of proteins that also allows their diverse set of functions is their ability to bind other molecules specifically and tightly.

Proteins also have structural or mechanical functions, such as actin and myosin in muscle and the proteins in the cytoskeleton, which form a system of scaffolding that maintains cell shape.

Other proteins are important in cell signaling, immune responses, cell adhesion, and the cell cycle. Proteins are also necessary diets, since humans cannot synthesize all the amino acids they need and must obtain essential amino acids from food.

Through the process of digestion, humans break down ingested protein into free amino acids that are then used in metabolism.

The best-known role of proteins in the cell is as enzymes, which catalyze chemical reactions. Enzymes are usually highly specific and accelerate only one or a few chemical reactions.

Enzymes carry out most of the reactions involved in metabolism, as well as manipulating DNA in processes such as DNA replication, DNA repair, and transcription.

Many proteins are involved in the process of cell signaling and signal transduction. Some proteins, such as insulin, are extracellular proteins that transmit a signal from the cell in which they were synthesized to other cells in distant tissues.

Antibodies are protein components of an adaptive immune system whose main function is to bind antigens, or foreign substances in the body, and target them for destruction.

Most microorganisms and plants can biosynthesize all 20 standard amino acids, while humans (including other animals) must obtain some of the amino acids from the diet.

The amino acids that an organism cannot synthesize on its own are referred to as essential amino acids.

Key enzymes that synthesize certain amino acids are not present in humans and animals. If amino acids are present in the environment, microorganisms can conserve energy by taking up the amino acids from their surroundings and down regulating their biosynthetic pathways.

In humans, amino acids are obtained through the consumption of foods containing protein. Ingested proteins are then broken down into amino acids through digestion, which typically involves denaturation of the protein through exposure to acid and hydrolysis by enzymes called proteases.

Some ingested amino acids are used for protein biosynthesis, while others are converted to glucose through gluconeogenesis, or fed into the citric acid cycle.

This use of protein as a fuel is particularly important under starvation conditions as it allows the body's own proteins to be used to support life, particularly those found in muscle. Amino acids are also an important dietary source of nitrogen.

Lipids

Lipids : are a group of naturally occurring molecules that include fats, sterols, fat-soluble vitamins (such as vitamins A, D, E, and K), monoglycerides, diglycerides, triglycerides, phospholipids, and others. The main biological functions of lipids include storing energy, signaling, and acting as structural components of cell membranes.

Although the term lipid is sometimes used as a synonym for fats, fats are a subgroup of lipids called triglycerides.

Lipids also encompass molecules such as fatty acids and their derivatives (including tri-, di-, monoglycerides, and phospholipids), as well as other sterol-containing metabolites such as cholesterol.

Although humans use various biosynthetic pathways to both break down and synthesize lipids, some essential lipids cannot be made this way and must be obtained from the diet.

The fatty acid structure is one of the most fundamental categories of biological lipids, and is commonly used as a building-block of more structurally complex lipids.

The carbon chain, typically between four and 24 carbons long, may be saturated or unsaturated, and may be attached to functional groups containing oxygen, halogens, nitrogen, and sulfur.

Lipid signaling is a vital part of the cell signaling. Lipid signaling may occur via activation of G protein-coupled or nuclear receptors, and members of several different lipid categories have been identified as signaling molecules and cellular messengers

One type of lipid is a potent messenger molecule involved in regulating calcium mobilization and cell growth, another type of fatty-acid derived eicosanoid involved in inflammation and immunity.

Certain lipids are known to be involved in signaling for the phagocytosis of apoptotic cells by which steroid hormones such as estrogen, testosterone and cortisol, which modulate a host of functions such as reproduction, metabolism and blood pressure.

Most of the fat found in food is in the form of triglycerides, cholesterol, and phospholipids. Some dietary fat is necessary to facilitate absorption of fat-soluble vitamins (A, D, E, and K) and carotenoids.

Humans have a dietary requirement for certain essential fatty acids, such as linoleic acid (an omega-6 fatty acid) and alpha-linolenic acid (an omega-3 fatty acid) because they cannot be synthesized from simple precursors in the diet.

A large number of studies have shown positive health benefits associated with consumption of omega-3 fatty acids on infant development, cancer, cardiovascular diseases, and various mental illnesses, such as depression, attention-deficit hyperactivity disorder, and dementia.

In contrast, it is now well-established that consumption of trans fats, such as those present in partially hydrogenated vegetable oils, are a risk factor for cardiovascular disease.

Carbohydrates

Carbohydrates : Comprising 75% of the biological world and 80% of all food intake for human consumption, the most common known human carbohydrate is Sucrose.

The simplest version of a carbohydrate is a monosaccharide which possesses the properties of carbon, hydrogen, and oxygen in a 1:2:1 ratio

Some type of Carbohydrates play key roles in the immune system, fertilization, preventing pathogenesis, blood clotting, and development.

Monosaccharides type of carbohydrates are the major source of fuel for metabolism, being used both as an energy source, glucose being the most important in nature, and in biosynthesis.

When monosaccharides are not immediately needed by many cells they are often converted to more space-efficient forms, often polysaccharides.

In many animals, including humans, this storage form is glycogen, especially in liver and muscle cells.

When not used immediately as an energy requirement for physical or bodily functions, it is stored in human body in different form for future utilization of energy.

Carbohydrates are a common source of energy in living organisms; however, no carbohydrate is an essential nutrient in humans.

Carbohydrates are not essential for the synthesis of other molecules. Humans are able to obtain 100% of their energy requirement from protein and fats.

Following a diet consisting of very low amounts of daily carbohydrate for several days will usually result in higher levels of blood ketone bodies than an isocaloric diet with similar protein content.

This relatively low level of ketones is commonly known as ketosis and is very often confused with the potentially fatal condition often seen in type 1 diabetics known as Diabetic ketoacidosis.

Somebody suffering Ketoacidosis will have much higher levels of blood ketone bodies along with high blood sugar, dehydration and electrolyte imbalance.

Nutritionists often refer to carbohydrates as either simple or complex. **However, the exact distinction between these groups can be ambiguous.**

The term complex carbohydrate was first used in the U.S. Senate Select Committee on Nutrition and Human Needs publication Dietary Goals for the United States

(1977) where it was intended to distinguish sugars from other carbohydrates which were perceived to be nutritionally superior.

However, the report put "fruit, vegetables and whole-grains" in the complex carbohydrate column, despite the fact that these may contain sugars as well as polysaccharides.

This confusion persists as today some nutritionists use the term complex carbohydrate to refer to any sort of digestible saccharide present in a whole food, where fiber, vitamins and minerals are also found as opposed to processed carbohydrates, which provide calories but few other nutrients.

The standard usage, however, is to classify carbohydrates chemically: simple if they are sugars (monosaccharides and disaccharides) and complex if they are polysaccharides (or oligosaccharides)

In any case, the simple vs. complex chemical distinction has little value for determining the nutritional quality of carbohydrates.

Water
Water : A major component of food is water, which can encompass anywhere from 50% in meat products to 95% in lettuce, cabbage, and tomato products.

It is also an excellent place for bacterial growth and food spoilage if it is not properly processed.

One way this is measured in food is by water activity which is very important in the shelf life of many foods during processing.

The human body contains from 55% to 78% water, depending on body size. To function properly, the body requires between one and seven liters of water per day to avoid dehydration; the precise amount depends on the level of activity, temperature, humidity, and other factors.

Most of this is ingested through foods or beverages other than drinking straight water.

It is not clear how much water intake is needed by healthy people, though most specialists agree that approximately 2 liters (6 to 7 glasses) of water daily is the minimum to maintain proper hydration. **Many ancient literature favors a lower consumption**, typically 1 liter of water for an average male, excluding extra requirements due to fluid loss from exercise or warm weather.

For those who have unhealthy kidneys, it is rather difficult to drink too much water, but especially in warm humid weather and while exercising, it is dangerous to drink too little.

People can drink far more water than necessary while exercising, however, putting them at risk of water intoxication (hyperhydration), which can be fatal.

The popular claim that "a person should consume eight glasses of water per day" seems to have no real basis in science. Similar misconceptions concerning the effect of water on weight loss and constipation have also been dispelled.

Till today there is no specific or scientific study that can define the balance of the above mentioned essential food (Proteins, Lipids, Carbohydrates and Water) combination can be the best with the use of Modern Medical Food Pyramid.

However in the Ancient Indian Healing literature and many other literatures around the world which deal in healing techniques it if very profound that the combination of the food that becomes the building block of the human body and system has to compliment the essential requirement of growth, repair and maintenance of the body composition.

Every human body with a different need would have different requirement of such basic building blocks.

No common diet chart of food pyramid can be a final declaration of human health, contrary to the popular belief.

No modern medical system can govern what is a essential FOOD Pyramid. In fact the use of modern Food Pyramid might be responsible for majority of Disorders prevalent in today's modern world.

Go to your basic, research the ancient literature on healing and wellbeing an numerous information and wisdom can be found all over the globe.

The balance for each and every individual human body cannot be dictated by a single modern medical chart. It is a ridiculous thought. However the common population has no Choice.

Its' been systematically fooled to believe that the modern Medical Food Pyramid used by doctors and Nutritionist around the world is the correct parameter.

Beware!!! Take care of your own bodies. Think is such Nutrition charts, Diet Charts and Food Pyramid could have been correct you would not need nutritionist and doctors to treat you with any other chemical and pharmaceutical substance.

Are you being fed with supplements and pills by any of such professional, take your body back from such torture.

I have seen many such doctors and nutritionist who have messed their own bodies with chemicals to show the world that they know what they are propagating, if fact themselves have not idea what the results of such pills and supplements would be in the distance future.

I have come across some many cases of Cancer and other serious disorders and suffering from people who have been taking fat loss pills, supplements, inject some sort of chemical and most important have been doing it in Secret or under some fitness guru.

I would only like to create awareness amongst all the people of the world, the common people, the naive people, the simple people, the population which is victimized in the name of healthcare.

Understand the difference between **sick-care and healthcare**.

Modern medical science is based on sickness and disorder, they have nothing for healthcare.

For health care you should first have a healthy body. Since the beginning of modern medical science there is nothing that has been done in Healthcare.

Even the father of medical science has clearly proclaimed.

Make food your Medicine . . . . else Medicine will become your food.

What is your choice . . . . Medicine or Food

Take a pick.

CHAPTER 5
NOT JUST POWER OF MIND, IT'S THE MIND

Believe you can and you're halfway there
—Theodore Roosevelt

Attention deficit disorder, clinic depression, Alzheimer's disease, autism, multiple personalities, anxiety, dementia, Parkinson's disease, schizophrenia. We have all heard of these brain disorders that cause loss of productivity, memory loss, and even death.

Upon further scientific inspection, it is obvious that the chemical imbalances in the brain are caused by diet, and stress more than anything else.

Instead of creating further imbalance within the brain by encouraging chemical concoctions, **it is time people recognized the natural methods to live happier and clearer in their everyday lives.**

If you think of your body as a car, plane, or machine of some sort then you might recognize just how important your diet is. The human body, and particularly the brain, is arguably one of the most complex and beautiful of any machines.

Like cars and planes, the human body needs fuel to provide power for our everyday lives. It is important to fill your body with the optimum fuel in order to see the most efficient results.

The brain is mostly comprised of fat and the primary way of maintaining a well-powered mind is through the fats that you eat.

As you may have heard, Omega 3 fatty acids are the healthiest type of fats that you can supply as fuel for your brain. The Omega 3 fatty acids help to build the cell membranes, balance your blood sugar, and increase brain-derived neurotrophic factor (BDNF) activity.

The BDNF activity is essential for supporting existing neurons and promoting neurogenesis. Perhaps most important for fixing the unbalanced brain is the Omega 3 fatty acids' ability to reduce the inflammation of the brain that is the cause of many brain disorders commonly treated with prescription pills.

The cell membranes in your body are also made of Omega 3 fatty acids, which are more fluid and allow connections to be made more freely. In comparison, trans-fats that comprise the largest percentage in our fry-happy culture are rigid and stiff. This has a direct correlation to slower and stiffer connections between cell membranes.

The food and drink that you ingest on a daily basis has a profound impact on the neuro-transmitters that influence your mood and allow your brain to function at a much higher capacity.

Maintaining a balance with these four important neuro-transmitters is necessary:
1. Dopamine
2. Seratonin
3. GABA (gamma-Aminobutyric acid)
4. Acetylcholine

Most common processed foods distort the balances in the body in the short-term and provide long-term problems for your body.

Many refined carbohydrates, such as grains, bread, pasta, and pizza, and refined sugars will temporarily increase the body's serotonin levels, but this prohibits the body from making and regulating levels efficiently over the long-term.

Even if you do not gain weight, abusing refined carbohydrates can lead to all types of brain imbalances and mood disorders.

The lopsided consumption of complex carbohydrates and sugar leads to many of the chemical imbalances that are treated with prescription drugs.

Consumption of carbs increase the abundance of cortisol in the body in addition to the short serotonin spike.

This increased cortisol activity is responsible for reducing the serotonin beyond balanced levels.

Similar to a deficit of neurotransmitters such as norepinephrine, epinephrine, and dopamine, this type of serotonin deficit can quickly create:
    -Depression
    -Appetite Cravings
    -Brain Fog
    -Low IQ
    -Anxiety
    -Panic Attacks
    -Insomnia
    -Eating disorders
    -Migraines
    -Ease of distraction or ADD

Millions of people walk around every day with some kind of neurotransmitter deficiency or suboptimal nerve cell communication. You've probably experienced at least one of these issues before, right? The good news is that you don't have to check yourself into a mental institution.

Interestingly, common depression and many other brain and mood disorders are treated with prescription drugs that are designed to artificially boost serotonin receptors in the brain. This however is not an answer.

If you remove certain foods, you will not have this problem in the first place!

Sometimes our environment can provide serious enough stimulus to make us anxious, nervous, or depressed.

Unfortunately, that is a part of life, but we can limit the bad moods and chronic depression with dietary habits, a healthy active regimen, and ample stress relief techniques.

Many degenerative and mood disorders have been linked to imbalances of chemicals within the brain, but **instead of correcting these problems through natural methods, prescription drugs are often the quick fix.**

In contrast to taking prescription drugs in order to balance our brains, it is important to search for and treat the root of the problem.

Correct and Balanced Diet is one of the most important parts of maintaining a balanced brain, but stress management can help balance the chemicals in your brain.

The greatest tragedy with the standard American diet which has become popular worldwide is the lack of nutrition given the energy consumed.

When one envisions malnourished individuals, it is of starving children in places in the world with a low socio-economic status. Just like these starving children, a majority of western populations are malnourished.

There are a number of essential vitamins, minerals, and nutrients that humans need to consume on a regular basis in order to maintain a balance of chemicals in the brain.

A lack of these nutrients leads to many of the mood disorders and degenerative diseases that are already common and on the rise like Depression Obesity, Diabetes, Thyroidism, Impotence, Infertility, PCOS, Sleep Disorders, Cholesterol, Chronic Heart Disorders etc.

The large majority of overweight or obese individuals are missing most, if not all, of the vital nutrients that they need in order to balance the chemicals in their brain.

It would be impractical and time consuming to go through the list of these nutrients.

Many of the long-latency deficiency diseases such as cancer, Alzheimer's, and autism are caused or exacerbated by a lack of a few major nutrients.

The body undergoes two processes called "methylation" and "sulfation," which are both relatively unknown but extremely important.

In order for your body to perform these processes, you must maintain a sufficient amount of folate (folic acid), vitamin B6 and **vitamin B12.**

Not only are all three of these necessary for proper methylation and sulfation, but they impact your mood as well.

An insufficient supply of folic acid has been linked to a large number of mood disorders.

This includes depression, anxiety, and a number of others one can resolve by eating sunflower seeds, beans, peas, lentils, or any leafy vegetable like spinach.

Similarly, vitamin B6, which can be found in many types of meat, regulates and produces serotonin in order to balance your brain.

Finally, lacking vitamin B12 can lead to significant depression, memory loss, and other brain problems. Unfortunately the amount of Vitamin B12 which is essential for human balanced nutrition is not present in the natural flora so it need to be taken from the fauna sources only.

Although many pills and supplement have been claiming Vitamin B12. According to my experiences only natural sources of vitamin B12 have made great and significant changes in my treatment of disorders like FAT Loss, Depression Obesity, Diabetes, Thyroidism, Impotence, Infertility, PCOS, Sleep Disorders, Cholesterol, Chronic Heart Disorders etc.

The human body can only utilize and synthesize the natural source of vitamin B12. All other unnatural, chemically produced sources are useless to cure any such disorders.

Many of the most important nutrients for your body are the ones that help you detoxify /remove toxic chemicals that will negatively affect your brain. In

Instead of getting these vital nutrients, most diets are laden with high carbohydrates and sugar.

One of the most dangerous culprits for disrupting the balances in your brain amongst others is high fructose corn syrup.

Modern media has caught on to the anti-high fructose corn syrup trend, but there is hardly any change in the change in the composition which primarily loads packed foods with this and other similar or similarly dangerous substances.

Thus general population should be careful in consuming these processed foods.

The amount of sugar that humans consume has exponentially increased since the Paleolithic era.

Even humans two hundred years ago ate a relatively small amount of sugar compared to modern man.

One of the causes for this is the invention and large-scale production of high fructose corn syrup.

Just looking in one cupboard of food in any modern household, anyone might find that over 55% of the processed items have such dangerous ingredient.

High fructose corn syrup is even in non-sweet foods, such as Ketchup.

The constant choice of food is the process of the mind.

The life script through which religion, tradition, culture, society, government, common knowledge . . . etc. are controlled and governed are prominent mind blocks towards better and balance health.

Natural and Balanced diet for hormonal balance is one of the most important ways to balance your brain and avoid mood and degenerative disorders that will not only decrease your productivity and efficiency, but can even lead to death.

Although you have probably spent years abusing your brain and your body, it is never too late to get a fresh start.

Reset your diet by taking steps to balance and select the natural building block of your cell from your daily food as you can.

The chemical balance in your brain can only be healthy when you prioritize things like sleep, relaxation, physical activity, and diet.

An epidemic of mood disorders and degenerative diseases have made millions of people miserable across the planet and modern prescription pills are not necessarily the answer.

The long-term effect of most medication is totally unknown.

They haven't been around long enough so there is no way of knowing how they affect your long-term health, the genes of the future generations and general wellbeing of humanity altogether.

Nonetheless, the large majority of cases can be solved by maintaining a good natural diet that is high in Omega 3 fatty acids and essential vitamins and minerals which you body synthesis from your daily natural food.

However, maintaining a balanced brain doesn't just come from diet alone. Try to maintain a sleep schedule that offers at least a very deep and sound sleep every single night.

The hormonal imbalance is governed by mind. There is no debate against. Thus its not just the power of your mind that you can alter your body to become healthy, bring back order and balance.

It is precisely the physical composition, strength and function of your brains which is the source of the power of your mind which holds the key to balance. Such balance, corrects a lot of disorder our people around the world are suffering from.

CHAPTER 6

BILLIONS OF US ARE LIVING ON TIPs

If your happiness depends on what somebody else does, I guess you do have a problem.

—Richard Bach

I remember the story of Titanic, it got hit by an iceberg. It is a scientific fact that between two to five percent of the iceberg is visible above the water surface. The remaining is below the water.

An iceberg is a large piece of freshwater ice that has broken off a glacier or an ice shelf and is floating freely in open water.

Typically only one-ninth of the volume of an iceberg is above water. Experts say usually 3% is visible to the mariners who are trained to spot an iceberg.

The shape of the underwater portion can be difficult to judge by looking at the portion above the surface.

This has led to the expression **"tip of the iceberg"**, for a problem or difficulty that is only a small manifestation of a larger problem.

The iceberg metaphor : Only 3 percent of the iceberg is seen as tip. Postulate—Important is hidden

A lot of mariners are very careful of the tip of iceberg. They are trained to identify and keep away from such visual clues. They steer clear and would never go near such tips.

On the contrary our world is filled with people who are never interested in the iceberg below and would crash themselves into any such tips. Such behavior has been synonymous with the popular culture and quick fix culture.

No one has time to understand the matter, they want tips, as if tips are going to solve their problems. To the contrary belief that one should be very careful of the tip.

For any problem, people jump for tips

Many a times these same tips devised to ease their pain become the reason of much greater pain in their live. And the blame games starts.

Nobody has time to understand the depth and weight of the any issue. Their behavior resembles the mariner who is naïve about the iceberg and sails towards the tip of an iceberg, hoping that it would be act as a stable anchor.

Nobody wants to understand the ninety seven percent of the iceberg. If ever they come to know the hidden gravity they would keep away from tips.

However our culture has blinded people and a majority live as if they want to crash into the three percent visible ice.

How can it possibly, be sensible?

Tips are also synonym as checklist of things to do.

This checklist can be good and useful is you know the subject.

This can be very dangerous when you don't know the subject

Half knowledge can be very dangerous; tips are just summary of whole meaning not even half knowledge.

People around the globe are speeding their life and depending on the tip culture to live their day to day life.

People around the world are crazy for tips on everything.
Weight Loss Tips
Weight Gain Tips
Living with Diabetes Tips

Living with Thyroid Tips
This tip and That Tips
10 Tips for this, 20 Tips for than, 100 Tips for something else.

The whole world is filled with people wanting short-cuts to overcome their pains and sufferings and equal number of us to provide such tips. However everyone get the short-cut to the opposite.

Our whole life is surrounded with tips for this and tips for that. Present culture of living on the tips has created a tsunami of misinformation and misdirection that cannot be undone so easily.

Whichever show I attend, whichever gathering I address, or wherever I see or meet people, people are hungry to get some tips. Their question is straight and simple **"Can you give us some tips on losing weight"**

Every time I come across this question on tips, I have to refrain myself from providing the most popular method of sharing information.

I ensure that I introduce them to their question. I challenge their thought process. I challenge them to open up to more serious issues than tips. See the gigantic problem below the tip.

When you don't know **WHY you are obese**, or why you have thyroid issues, or sleep disorder or diabetes etc. **How on earth can any tip from anyone in the world would help.**

Such Tips are going the complicate your situation more than what it is today. Make your life more miserable.

You will create your own perception about the underlining knowledge and start questioning the authenticity of the process.

The media in itself is not responsible; however it cannot be a subject of ignorance and innocence.

Every day they bombard the general population with so many tips from so many sources, creating chaos around any subject matter.

Yet I say, You cannot blame anyone. You cannot blame the media, or any other source.

We as humans are the true culprits of this major chaos.

We get what we desire and deserve. If we are suffering because of the pill culture then do not forget we humans desired it in the past

Similarly, if today, we as humans desire to get rid to the pills **we certainly can and we certainly will**.

Today, if we want to remove pain from our life **we can**. The journey requires a traveler. You can't reach the destination without taking the journey.

Natural cure has the answers. Search for appropriate places, do your own discovery, research and you will find the solutions of your chronic pains and suffering.

If you still don't get your answers, contact Dr. Lall's Natural Care and Wellness Centre, we always provide the right direction.

We as a common population just need to understand the difference between Disease and Disorder and choose the course of action to make well of our health and wellbeing.

Because **modern medicine refuses to really acknowledge this single central fact**, it cannot cure us or our children of what ails us in this modern day and age.

So what can actually cure us in these modern days? **The main cure for illness, which was first written of by Hippocrates—the father of modern medicine!—is food! It's true!**

Making wise decisions about what we put into our bodies can change that internal landscape dramatically so that we no longer experience symptoms of disease and illness, because there wont be any illness.

Hippocrates himself said : Make food your medicine or medicine will become your food.

To find out more about how you can use wholesome, nutritious food to heal your own body and those of your children, Reach out to Dr. Lall's Nature Care Clinic which gives plenty of information on specific ways you can heal yourself and your children through making smart choices that can change their internal landscape for the better.

Free yourself from the temptation of the Tips Culture and you will find your path. We can guide you.

The traveler still has to travel alone to reach destination.

CHAPTER 7
Clearopathy Treatment
ITS SIMPLE, NOT EASY

Life is really simple, but we insist on making it complicated.

—Confucius

The Pareto principle somehow reflect in many aspect of our life . . . . 80 % of people are governed by 20% people etc. 20% is responsible for 80% of the resources, etc. etc.

20% of imbalance in the human body is responsible for 80% of the disorders. This 20% according to Dr. Lall is the issues related to Endocrine System and particularly their imbalance in managing the hormonal system.

If only body needs to be corrected 80 percent nutrition and 20 percent physical workout can help. This is the reason most of the animal based research do not apply to human.

The results of such research fail when utilized in real living human out of any laboratory condition.

Human are not subordinate animals of lower level with undeveloped brains.

Human are very much a thinking species and intelligent being, which have a perspective for each and everything around and the events that occurs in its life.

So when we are dealing with humans, we cannot be blinded with the fact that the human has something very important and very dominant controlling and managing them.

A very important function, that plays a very strong role in its own survival or destruction. Yes, i.e. **The human Mind.**

More about The 80:16:4 Formula
The 80:16:4 Formula thereby represents 80% Psychological Corrections 16% Nutrition Corrections and 4% Workout Corrections.

This formula is not just for Permanent Weight Loss but also to correct many Hormonal Disorders like Diabetes, Thyroid, Obesity, Inflammation Disorders and many more.

Most of these Disorders happen due to continuous distortion of food composition for years and imbalanced lifestyle habits culminating into regular high level of STRESS.

In my 12 years in the Freedom from medicine & weight loss field I have identified 16 rules which will make the biggest difference in people's weight and health.

Understanding the 16 Rules of this programs is the key to take total control over your life and health. To know about this 16 Rules do not forget to book you own copy when the book "Why We Fail" gets published.

What is great about this program is the approach. We do not focus on any eating habit or workout regime so the risk of getting overwhelmed is very very low.

The biggest mistake I see people make is trying to change too many eating habits at once so they can lose weight fast or incorporating too many workout regimes trying to accelerate the results.

As I have said before, trying to make too many changes at once is the best way to burn out regardless of the results you achieve.

For the people who want to lose weight fast, I have one question? What is the point of losing weight fast, if you are going to regain it all back again?

Wouldn't you rather take a few extra months to lose the weight the right way and never have to worry about your weight again?

Dr. LALL's FREEDOM FROM MEDICINE Programs for : PERSONAL, COMMUNITY & CORPORATES.

The FREEDOM FROM MEDICINE Program is a program focused on the daily dependence on medicine for various disorders.

Coaching of mind in the public or group scenario open door to treatment and therapy that was never experimented and tried in the are of Weight Loss and Drug Loss.

The Attention Abundance therapy is a process oriented treatment in Weight Loss and Drug Loss. It is more than helping people to decide what to change (ie, eating, activity, and thinking habits); it is helping them identify how to change.

Thus, once a goal is specified, patients are encouraged to examine factors that will facilitate or hinder goal achievement.

Cases in which the desired behavior is not implemented, problem-solving skills are used to identify new strategies to overcome barriers.

In this view, successful weight management is based on skills that can be learned and practiced, in the same manner that an individual can learn to play the piano through frequent practice.

Skill power, not will power, is the key to success.

The 80:16:4 Formula Revealed to groups in the community.

The best and easiest way to make lasting changes in your eating habits so you can lose weight or drug permanently and improve your health in the process achieving Wellness for life

There are plenty of good diet books and programs in the market today, yet we are still losing the weight loss battle.

There are a couple of reasons why most diets fail (fail to keep the weight off long term) but the main reason is that they fail to apply change into someone's life without overwhelming them.

They don't explain to the reader **why we fail the battle against Weight loss, Hormonal Imbalance, Diabetes, Thyroid, Inflammation Disorders, Impotence, Infertility etc.**

They don't tell why we develop imbalance food habits, how to best eliminate bad eating habits and choices and how to develop good ones.

They expect that people can just get up one morning and start eating a completely different way than they are used to doing.

FREEDOM FROM MEDICINE Program is a Program designed for the **Mind** which rules every aspect of our lifestyle and choices. Diet word itself comes from root word in Greek actually means Lifestyle or life choices.

They wrongly assume that once somebody starts seeing results they are motivated to stick with their diet program.

WRONG!

If results were enough to motivate, then why can't most people stick with the diet that helped them lose the weight and why do they end up regaining all the weight?

The fact is the best results in the world will not keep you motivated if you achieved those results through a method that overwhelmed you, and I think there is plenty of proof.

At **Dr. Lall's Nature Care Clinic (which Uses Naturopathy, Psychology, Nutrition, Diet, Pain & Fitness Expertise)** we have developed a very simple program to help our clients make permanent changes in their dietary (lifestyle) habits.

With our approach, we don't just teach our clients what foods to eat and what foods to avoid. We show them step by step how to best eliminate their bad eating habits providing the secrets why we have them at the first place.

At the same time develop good eating habits.

This program has been a great success with our clients at our Clinic and community Programs focusing Women support groups and we now offer the same program to corporations to help their employees lose weight, lose pills/drugs/medicine and improve their health.

A nice side effect of healthy employees is that they get sick less often which is good for them and for the Community. Our program carries a very low risk of burnout and is very easy to follow.

How the Community Program works
It is very simple. **Twice a Month,** Dr. Lall, the inventor of Clearopathy, address the group at their location for about 60 minute.

At the meeting, Dr. Lall discusses matter which is not available in the common knowledge domain, research and results which are not published in the leading media, however are very important for individual health and wellness.

He picks the thought process and other habit that the group will work on for the next 15 days only. This program works for a single group for 12 months. 2 hours per month at a time.

The lifestyle and eating habits are chosen in the order of importance. Each participant will receive a small guide book with the **lifestyle habit and thought process** that they should be working on. The booklet will help the participant stay on track with the application of the lifestyle habit.

The Program Achieves its target when the participants understand the reasons **WHY** it is what it is today, only then they begin to apply the new lifestyle habit into their lives, there are always obstacles that get in the way.

The weekly meeting is the time to bring up any obstacles faced by any team member during the past 7 days.

These obstacles are understood by everyone and the whole group provides the much needed attention the individual raising the obstacles faced.

All discuss the reasons WHY such thing happened. This creates an environment of Attention Abundance for any individual who had been struggling in the past seven days.

Many obstacles they will face, other people before them have already faced and we have come up with solutions. Once in a while, new obstacles come up that no one else has faced before.

If that is the case, Dr. Lall will sit with the person and teams and help them come up with a solution that best works for them.

The focus of this formula is to achieve the **target result within 12 months** and all together within the group. The motto is not to leave anyone behind. Everyone tracks the progress of each other together along with Dr. Lall

Main Benefit of this program

1. Because weight loss will be achieved though **permanent changes** into people's lifestyle habits, it will be easy for people to keep the weight off on completion of the program.

2. Because we work on exposing the **Root Cause of various habit at a time**, people will have a much easier time sticking with this program and actually losing the weight they want.

3. You do not need to do this program for the rest of your life in order to keep the weight off. Once people have established the lifestyle habits they need and have lost the weight they want, and they do it **within the specified 12 months and see results on their own**.

4. This is not a diet. **This is an Eat2Beat Disorders Program.** With this program people will **not have to count calories,** weigh their food, or count points. They will simply learn **Why to eat** for the right reasons again.

5. People will not just learn what dietary changes they will need to make, but will also learn how to apply those changes in their life without getting overwhelmed.

6. With this program people will not just loss weight, they will also improve their health, can come out of Diabetes, Thyroid etc. which means less cost on sickness treatment per year.

InvestmentThe cost is only a fraction of what you might be spending on medication for your present ailment. The cost is nearly equivalent to the gymnasium fee per month for any individual participant.

The participants take care of the investment and become more responsible for themselves. We encourage the community leaders to promote the program for the benefit of their Residents.

Each participant becomes the part of One Team. Each Team size would be not be less than 50. If your Community has more than 50 people who would like to participate in our programs, we can create more groups/Teams if required, else larger the group greater the Abundance of Attention and amazing is the effect of the Dr. Lall's Attention Abundance Therapy.

> *—Be Healthy by Choice, Not by Chance!!!*
> *—Dr. S. Lall*

REFERENCES

1) Endocrinology: Tissue Histology. University of Nebraska at Omaha. http://www.unomaha.edu/hpa/endocrinehistology.html

2) Colorado State University-Biomedical Hypertextbooks-Somatostatin http://www.vivo.colostate.edu/hbooks/pathphys/endocrine/index.html

3) Silverman, Marni N.; Pearce, Brad D.; Biron, Christine A.; Miller, Andrew H. (1 March 2005). "Immune Modulation of the Hypothalamic-Pituitary-Adrenal (HPA) Axis during Viral Infection". Viral Immunology

4) Kaushansky K (May 2006). "Lineage-specific hematopoietic growth factors". N Engl J Med. 354 (19): 2034-45. doi:10.1056/NEJMra052706. PMID 16687716.

5) Pentikäinen V, Erkkilä K, Suomalainen L, Parvinen M, Dunkel L (May 2000). "Estradiol acts as a germinal cell survival factor in the human testis in vitro". J Clin Endocrinol Metab. 85 (5): 2057-67. doi:10.1210/jc.85.5.2057. PMID 10843196.

6) Hould F, Fried G, Fazekas A, Tremblay S, Mersereau W (1988). "Progesterone receptors regulate gallbladder motility". J Surg Res 45 (6): 505-12. doi:10.1016/0022-4804(88)90137-0. PMID 3184927.

7) Massaro D, Massaro GD (2004). "Estrogen regulates pulmonary alveolar formation, loss, and regeneration in mice". American Journal of Physiology. Lung Cellular and Molecular Physiology

   Bortolotti, M. and Barbara, L. (1988). Interdigestive gastroduodenal motor activity in subjects with increased gastric acid secretion. Digestion 41: 156-160.

8) Frühbeck G (July 2004). "The adipose tissue as a source of vasoactive factors". Curr Med Chem Cardiovasc Hematol Agents 2 (3): 197-208. doi:10.2174/1568016043356255. PMID 15320786.

9) Sherwood, L. (1997). Human Physiology: From Cells to Systems. Wadsworth Pub Co

10) Turnbull, AV; Rivier, CL (1999 Jan). "Regulation of the hypothalamic-pituitary-adrenal axis by cytokines: actions and mechanisms of action.". Physiological reviews 79 (1): 1-71. PMID 9922367.

11) O'Connor, TM; O'Halloran, DJ; Shanahan, F (2000 Jun). "The stress response and the hypothalamic-pituitary-adrenal axis: from

molecule to melancholia.". QJM : monthly journal of the Association of Physicians 93 (6): 323-33. doi:10.1093/qjmed/93.6.323. PMID 10873181.

12) Sarkar, C; Basu, B; Chakroborty, D; Dasgupta, PS; Basu, S (2010 May). "The immunoregulatory role of dopamine: an update". Brain, behavior, and immunity 24 (4): 525-8. doi:10.1016/j. bbi.2009.10.015. PMC 2856781. PMID 19896530.

13) Tsigos, C; Chrousos, GP (2002 Oct). "Hypothalamic-pituitary-adrenal axis, neuroendocrine factors and stress". Journal of psychosomatic research 53 (4): 865-71. doi:10.1016/S0022-3999(02)00429-4. PMID 12377295.

14) Andrews, Nancy C. (30 April 2004). "Anemia of inflammation: the cytokine-hepcidin link". Journal of Clinical Investigation 113 (9): 1251-1253. doi:10.1172/JCI21441. PMC 398435. PMID 15124013.

15) DICKHOFF, WALTON W.; DARLING, DOUGLAS S. (1 January 1983). "Evolution of Thyroid Function and Its Control in Lower Vertebrates". Integrative and Comparative Biology 23 (3): 697-707. doi:10.1093/icb/23.3.697.

16) Hartenstein, V (2006 Sep). "The neuroendocrine system of invertebrates: a developmental and evolutionary perspective". The Journal

of endocrinology 190 (3): 555-70. doi:10.1677/
joe.1.06964. PMID 17003257.

17) "Mortality and Burden of Disease Estimates for
WHO Member States in 2002" (xls). World Health
Organization. 2002.

18) Endo K, Matsumoto T, Kobayashi T, Kasuya Y,
Kamata K (February 2005). "Diabetes-related
changes in contractile responses of stomach
fundus to endothelin-1 in streptozotocin-induced
diabetic rats".

19) GALTON, VALERIE ANNE (1 January 1988).
"The Role of Thyroid Hormone in Amphibian
Development". Integrative and Comparative
Biology 28 (2): 309-318. doi:10.1093/icb/28.2.309.

20) Kasper (2005). Harrison's Principles of
Internal Medicine. McGraw Hill. p. 2074. ISBN
0-07-139140-1.

21) Chronic Hunger and Obesity Epidemic; Eroding
Global Progress, World Watch Institute, March 4,
2000

22) Childhood overweight and obesity, WHO, August
22, 2010

23) Prevalence of overweight & obesity for
males over 15, 2002-2010, WHO International
Comparisons, November 19, 2010

24) Blair Golson, America's Eating Disorder, Alternet. org, April 19, 2006

25) http://www.who.int/features/qa/49/en/index.html

26) http://www.euro.who.int/en/health-topics/ noncommunicable-diseases/obesity

http://www.telegraph.co.uk/health/3290602/ Dependence-day-the-rise-of-pill-culture.html

27) http://www.hhs.gov/